eye & ivy

by Michael L. Stone

Stepping Stone Sports, LLC.

Photo credit: Erik Stenbakken

Cover co-design: Dave Meas

Additional photos of Michael Stone by Betsy Bulkley

Book design: Roche Design

ISBN 978-1-4276-4674-3

Eye Envy was created in a larger font size of 16 points. A 16-point font is actually smaller than what most people with low vision find easily readable. For example, my computer is set to a minimum of 18 points. I gave the font size much thought and angst about writing a book intended for those with low vision anything less than they could read. It is my hope that those who are fully sighted gain some understanding that although the font used in this book might seem enormous to their eyes, it is actually on the small side for the millions of others affected with sight impairments.

dedication

This book is dedicated to all those who have chosen to devote their lives to helping others achieve the most rewarding lives possible by going that extra step for those who really need it — whatever *it* might be. To those who grow weary from the challenges life has thrown their way: May they find peace.

To my beloved parents, who have given me the two greatest gifts this world has ever given me: my two brothers. To my beloved brothers, who have shown me what love really means. Life without you would not be the same. Your support from the day you both entered this world has gone well beyond what a big brother could ever ask. You have given me light when the light just wasn't so bright.

In loving memory of Norman Silverman, my grandfather, who hid his true struggles of vision loss from macular degeneration.

table of contents

eye envy

acknowledgments

Eye Envy was always meant to be a guide to those who really needed someone to relate to, as well as to learn more about the devastating effects of retinal degenerative diseases. *Those* is defined as anyone affected by the rapid or gradual loss of vision. Getting through life is challenging enough without having a disability or having a disabled loved one. We can't possibly succeed in making the most of the adventures life offers us without help from the people who love us most.

It would be near impossible to acknowledge

everyone who has inspired and *been there* for me. I am certain that no words exist that can express my gratitude for the support these special people continue to provide me. For those of you that I missed in this section, please know that my gratitude extends beyond just what is in print.

My parents, Barbara and Joel Stone: I know we sometimes lack the words that express our feelings about the challenges life may cast upon us. I also know that the vision-loss challenges both my brother and I face have weighed heavily on you. Your continued support to raise awareness and funds in an effort to find cures and treatments for these diseases has such deep meaning in my heart that I simply cannot thank you enough.

My family: Lily, Sari, Ori, Summer, Ryder, David and Yvette, Russell and Shelly … enough said!

My friends: Anyone who knows me also knows that I don't use the term "friend" lightly. You know who you are. Thank you for all of your support.

Wes Hobson: From a guy I met at the pool in my early days of triathlon to one of my best friends. Your frequent jests with me during our runs — saying "Don't give me any of this 'I can't see' crap! You see just fine" — are quite often exactly what I need. It's difficult not to laugh when I'm putting every ounce of energy into not falling. I am so grateful for you not letting me give in to those *dark* moments.

Michael Balaban: For over 20 years of loyal friendship and for following me halfway around the world to remind me to "dig deep!"

Kimberley Robottom: Love comes in the most unexpected ways. You light my heart in the purest way. Your strength gives me strength and your smile warms my heart. Thank you for never giving up — on us both.

Ann and Felicity Robottom: For teaching me that *family* can be expanded, no matter what the physical distance is. Your support and love have kept me going right from the beginning of our relationship. You will always be the "Hell on Wheels Gang."

Gordon and Lulie Gund: For showing *us* how to help *us* help ourselves. You redefine what it means to have hope.

Dr. Gerald Fishman: For filling in the missing piece that had plagued me for over 35 years.

Dr. Coleman Kraff: For never giving up on finding an answer to why I "just can't see better." For helping make a dream come true.

Ivy Koger, Jared Berg, Brad Seng, Will Laughlin, and Ryan Ignatz For being my "eyes" and guiding me to some of the most rewarding experiences of my life. You were also my teachers and helped introduce to me to such a wider reality. I am forever grateful. Ivy and Jared, those were some of the greatest experiences of my life — so far!

Ryan Van Praet: Another visually impaired

athlete struggling to adapt to the evolution of his racing and sharing this transitional experience with me, even when it was causing him the greatest of pain. You give this book very special meaning.

Matt Miller: The fully sighted founder of the C Different Foundation, who does his part to make dreams a reality.

Janet Stenerson: Someone who was there for me in my darkest of moments and really knows the meaning of love, loss and the healing powers of chicken soup.

Makenna Hobson: For your continued love and making your sometimes lonely next-door friend feel not so lonely!

Michael and Wink Jackson (Zeal Optics): Thank you for believing in me and making the best, most versatile eyewear on the market that allows me to do the activities I love most.

I'd like to thank those who directly helped me

with *Eye Envy*, whether it was part of my research or just support: Roman Mica, David and Lisa Young, Dr. Tim Schoen, Bill Schmidt, Ben Shaberman, Jeremy Block, Aaron Bishop, Dave Meas, Mary Jarrett and Judith Holding.

Lastly, all those who participated in the initial phase of the Race to Cure Blindness and getting it off the ground: Sally Mitchell, Christina Donatelli, Kristine Amendola, Stacy Fass, Adam Zucco, Susan Davis, Michael Kelly, Erica Shifflett, AJ and Courtney Johnson, Kay Stolcis, Craig Howie, Sue, Graham and Ryann Fraser, Scott Fliegelman, Jen Szabo, Carolyn Rickard, Cathy Koger (your continued push was exactly what I needed), and of course "Kahuna" Dave Nicholas (from Xterra), Barry and Jodee Siff and Lynn Christianson.

foreword

"The intricate inner workings of our bodies are easy to take for granted. It is when we become challenged medically that we pause, seek out help, and hopefully find resolution to the problem. Michael knew at a young age something was amiss with his vision. Years of educational struggle ensued, sprinkled with visits to numerous medical professionals who prescribed lots of contact lenses, which did not seem to alleviate the visual problems. A diagnosis of cone-rod dystrophy, a disease that would eventually render him blind, was the answer. Most people would become incapacitated when presented with this news. Not Michael. When faced with the prospect of losing his vision, Michael became an advocate for the blind as a fundraiser, a student and a mentor. Instead of shrinking away from activities that would scare people with excellent vision, Michael sought them out — he mountain bikes on difficult terrain, cross country skis, and runs through lava fields. This book is a culmination of his journey and will hopefully aid those dealing with losing their vision."

Joanna Zeiger, Ph.D.,
epidemiologist, professional triathlete,
Olympian and founder of *Fast at Forty*

"It is my honor to be included in this book not only because I am Michael's brother, but because I also suffer from cone-rod dystrophy. I realize how fortunate I was that when I was diagnosed in 2007, Michael had already begun the process of learning about the disease and how to cope with it. Without a book like this one, Michael had to look to many other resources to find information and ways to deal with this impairment. So many people are left in the dark on how to proceed with life knowing they have a life-altering disease. *Eye Envy* eases the pain and acts as a guide and resource to finding information and bringing the visually impaired community closer together. I believe this book is an invitation to a larger open forum of people across the world to share their feelings and experiences. The vision landscape is constantly in motion with new diagnoses and research, and trying to find answers can be daunting. *Eye Envy* helps those who cannot find the answers they are looking for from their doctors. I speak for myself, and our entire family, when I say how proud we are of Michael and his accomplishment."

Russell Stone,
Michael's brother

"Having clear vision for the majority of your life, only to have it indiscriminately and incurably diminish over a lengthy period of time, *could* be an inexorably depressing feeling. The subconscious might whisper that the best part of your life is over. In the book *Eye Envy,* Michael

Stone rejects this thought. In fact, he and others have made their lives even more productive than they probably would have been without a retinal degenerative disease. For instance, would Michael have ever done 10 Ironman triathlons and 25 Half-Ironmans in six consecutive years if he *hadn't* received a diagnosis that would eventually take the majority of his sight? He followed these athletic achievements by recently competing in the Xterra World Triathlon Championships (swim, *mountain bike*, off-road-run triathlon. Being a consistent training partner of Michael's, I have watched his vision deteriorate and am amazed by his determination to adapt to the disease while achieving such major accomplishments.

"The stories of Michael and other champions in this book inspire you to get off of the couch and expand your comfort zone, not letting life pass in an ordinary fashion. In laymen's language, Michael explains this disease so you have a better understanding of what is affecting the lives of over 10 million people in the United States. Although a cure has not been found, there is hope as hundreds of medical professionals are diligently working on putting the puzzle of genetics together for a solution. Knowing Michael for over a decade, as a friend and mentor, I have been inspired by his fortitude, charisma and drive not to let this disease slow him down. A cure will come."

Wes Hobson,
former professional triathlete, whose numerous wins and honors, such as "Triathlete of the Year" from the United States Olympic Committee, highlight his 12-year career and over 220 triathlons

introduction

What a difficult statement I have to make on a daily basis. "I am *not blind*! Well — not yet, but I'm *going* blind."

I am what is called visually impaired, or a person with low vision — the proper nomenclature of the day is so confusing that even I don't know how to refer to myself. I was not born blind, but have gradually been losing my eyesight since I was a child.

My friend Madeline Cohen, who has Usher's syndrome, began the fundraising letter for her annual vision walk with this statement: "I am *still* going blind!" Even I had to read this several times before the meaning really penetrated. Both Madeline and I have retinal degenerative diseases. It seems every few months there is something else that we used to be able to see but cannot anymore. It's a gradual process, though for some the process can be rapid.

I tell people, "Sorry, I don't see very well," but this broad statement doesn't really explain my situation. And although there are many sights and images that I miss, I still see more than many others who also have retinal degenerative diseases and are legally blind.

Retinal Degenerative Diseases (RDDs) is a term that covers a large number of rare conditions that cause severe vision loss and, eventually, blindness. Most people don't really understand what I am talking about when I talk about RDDs. It isn't until I say, "Have you heard of macular degeneration?" that the average person starts to "get" it. Many people ask, "Isn't that what that guy in Las Vegas,

Steve Wynn, has?" And I reply, "Close — he has retinitis pigmentosa, but they're different diseases. You might say they are cousins."

Even then, they still have very little idea of what these diseases are, though they affect over 10 million Americans and many millions more worldwide.

Retinal degenerative diseases include retinitis pigmentosa (RP), Stargardt's disease or Stargardt's macular dystrophy, macular degeneration, cone-rod dystrophy, Leber's congenital amaurosis (LCA), and Usher's syndrome (the degenerative process of losing both sight and hearing), to name a few. Many of us diagnosed with one of these diseases are not aware of what is happening at first. But over time, we gradually lose more ability to see, and each day becomes a greater challenge. Often, our eye doctors struggled to understand why they could not improve our vision when the retinal problems began to affect us. It's difficult to diagnose these diseases, and frustrating for everyone involved.

Our experiences are different from those of people who are born blind. Those of us who are losing our eyesight (whether from a young age, gradually over years, or rapidly during midlife) have relied on sightedness to orient us in the world. We face different challenges than people who never had sight and developed their other senses from birth.

Most people assume that being blind or gradually becoming blind means living in darkness. However, for many of us it means going into extreme lightness. A 2009 *Boulder Magazine* article about me aptly described my experience with cone-rod dystrophy as "Fade to White." In addition, we who have an RDD have blind spots, shapes and colors that block our vision in the center or on the periphery, and the blocking of our vision gets progressively worse over time.

We are fortunate that people have opened up their lives to the world to help spread some awareness of diseases that cause the loss of sight. For the majority of people, however, there is still little understanding or awareness of what these diseases are and how their symptoms affect those who have them.

Why this book?

I just love it when someone sees me struggling to read and says, "Dude, get some glasses!" or "Did you leave your reading glasses at home?" Oh yes, that just warms my heart. When I explain my disease and why simply wearing eyeglasses won't help, they usually say, "Then you should have Lasik surgery." Apparently I don't explain the situation well, or they just can't comprehend that this is a disease that *for now* can't be fixed by surgery or technology. Needless to say, it is exhausting to explain my problem every day, and it just makes me that much more fervent to find a cure.

I am hopeful that readers of this book will see why they should help spread awareness of diseases that cause vision loss so that we can treat *and cure* these diseases. The problem is that cures won't fund themselves. All of these diseases are what are called "orphan diseases." They don't receive the attention other diseases do. It is easy to understand how people might perceive diseases of the eye as not life threatening. I once shared that sentiment and would naively refer to my own disease as "life altering." But as you read on, you'll find that this is far from the case. These diseases are indeed quite life threatening.

In fact, I am convinced that when we cure blindness, we also will cure a plethora of other diseases. Doctors and scientists researching cures for Parkinson's disease and Alzheimer's have unanimously told me that the treatments and cures are very much linked to those for RDDs.

This book contains stories of people who have RDDs. It also features the families of those directly affected by RDDs and tells what they are doing to make the lives of their loved ones with RDDs just a little easier.

I pray that readers who are affected by one or more retinal degenerative diseases will be able to learn from these stories. I know how difficult it has been for my family and friends to watch me lose my vision and deal with the challenges it has created. Perhaps reading a book such as this one would have helped them, as well as me, when I was first diagnosed with cone-rod dystrophy.

In fact, even people who have vision difficulties that have nothing to do with retinal disease — people with corneal problems, for example — can relate to many of the stories in this book. Even though our disease treatments differ, our experiences coping with vision changes and their associated physical and emotional challenges can be similar.

I also hope that teachers will gain greater sensitivity when coping with a student who may seem to be "acting up" or otherwise causing a disturbance in the classroom. That student just might have a secret that not even he or she is aware of yet. I can't emphasize this enough. What happens in the classroom can change a person's life! Several people in this book, including me, were told by their teachers, "Stop faking, you can see just fine. You are just trying to get attention."

For example, my sixth-grade reading teacher was told to move me out of remedial reading into a higher-level class after testing determined that I was misplaced. The teacher was not happy. He said, "I am being forced to move you up a couple of levels. I don't think you deserve it, and I think you will fail." What a horrible thing to say to an 11-year-old child. My slow reading was not the result of not being able to decode words; it was due to my vision problems. I just wasn't aware that was the case.

I hope that each person reading this who has a disease like mine will feel a little less alone in the world. There are millions of people worldwide who can relate these stories to their own experiences. And, as you will read in Chapter 15 ("Science and Hope"), cures and treatments are imminent. You will read about the various clinical trials that are in different stages that have had incredibly positive results. I can only hope that readers will find solace in this information.

During my research, I learned how isolated those affected by losing their sight can feel. Giving up one's driver's license is devastating, as is losing the ability to navigate each day's most "insignificant" events after years of never having to think twice about such things. As the disease progresses, many people feel less and less able to go out into the world, essentially becoming isolated in their own homes.

It is remarkable how often I hear from those affected that they share the same fears as me. In the last month, for example, I heard it from more than 30 people. Some of these fears include being afraid to blink, that when my eyes open again I won't be able to see. This of course includes going to sleep. I went months with what felt like no sleep, enduring the fear that if I went to sleep, I wouldn't have sight when I awoke. Then there are the nightmares that go with these fears. The nightmares feel very real. It is a recurring nightmare that I was awaking to no sight at all. There are also the dreams that I would have perfect sight only to actually awake to the reality of no positive change in sight. This is not the way to start one's day. As I said, I was not alone with these experiences.

Imagine that your normal routine of getting dressed, making breakfast, reading your favorite newspaper, getting your kids off to school and heading off to work by car, bike, bus or foot slowly becomes difficult because your vision is "not quite right." You make an appointment to see your ophthalmologist, and after what may be months — or years — of medical tests, you learn that doing those seemingly insignificant tasks isn't so insignificant. Day by day, you are losing your sight. One day, you will no longer see your reflection in the mirror. You'll lose the ability to see your kids' faces; you won't be able to help get their breakfast or take them to school or see their latest performances or report cards. I assure you that I understate the effects of these retinal nightmares and their progression, but you can perhaps get a little understanding of what it's like.

Eye Envy picks up after that visit to the ophthalmologist's office where you've finally received the diagnosis that you have a disease that will lead to blindness. You might say this book offers "one-stop shopping" to help you find your way. I want you to feel inspired, comforted and encouraged as you read it. At the same time, you will be pleased to know that most of the proceeds of *Eye Envy* will go to researching cures and treatments for these diseases. Some of the proceeds will also go to helping visually challenged people find their passion and a way to express it in the form of athletics or art, for example.

I was only diagnosed in late 2003, but my story starts some 33 years earlier, as I struggled throughout my life with vision problems that I thought were "normal." I now know that there are millions of people who share my struggle. When I think about my challenges as a young person, I'm saddened to realize that life might have been very different and certainly easier had the doctors been able to diagnose my problem earlier. It is common for people with retinal degenerative diseases to be misdiagnosed, though an accurate diagnosis generally doesn't take as long as in my case! As you will see, many of the people featured in the book were misdiagnosed at one point. I learned that it was common for people with these diseases to be "missed" because RDDs were confused with behavioral disorders.

The courageous people featured in *Eye Envy* have graciously shared their stories to show the world that although they have challenges to overcome, they have accomplished extraordinary things while maintaining ordinary lives.

Much of the proceeds from the book will go to the Foundation Fighting Blindness (visit www. blindness.org for details). As far as I know, FFB is the only foundation dedicated to researching cures and treatments for *all* retinal degenerative diseases. The Foundation gives everyone hope. Why do I say "everyone"? Because many of you or your loved ones reading this book might have relatively perfect vision today, only to find out during midlife that you suddenly struggle to see. This is the case for most of us who have these diseases.

I am certain that it pains the doctor who delivers the bad news that you are going to go blind to say, "There is nothing I can do to help you. Good luck." Doctors would love to say, "I know it is hard and you are frightened, but we can treat this." Everything that researchers are doing suggests that a cure and/or treatments are imminent; they just need our support. As mentioned above, this book would be incomplete without a discussion of where the research is currently. You will find it in the "Science and Hope" chapter (Chapter 15), as well as on the FFB website.

In the chapters that follow, you will read about people of all ages, backgrounds and occupations who have managed to overcome their challenges. They are extraordinary people who do ordinary things. They include lawyers, artists, athletes, mothers, fathers, reporters, writers and businesspeople who achieved their personal career goals with limited or no use of their vision. They have shared their secrets to their road to healing as they met the challenges of continuous vision loss, and in many cases both vision and hearing loss. In most cases these people have learned to simultaneously excel in many different career and extracurricular fields.

I am inspired by many other people with diseases that have taken their sight. Some of them have written their own stories, including Marla Runyan, an Olympic runner who has Stargardt's disease; Eric Weihenmayer, the blind mountaineer who has summited Mount Everest and now leads other visually challenged people on mountain-climbing ascents around the world; and the famous tenor Andrea Bocelli! I strongly encourage you to read their stories. Marla's book was the first that I read when I decided to actually try to relate to other athletes who had retinal degenerative diseases.

Of course, there are many other courageous people who have an RDD who are now public figures, such as the governor of New York, David Patterson, the first legally blind governor in the U.S. He has been very open about his condition. The same holds true for the former San Francisco Mayor, Willie Brown. I recently had the pleasure of meeting Mayor Brown at the 2010 FFB Dining in the Dark event in San Francisco. This event is exactly what it sounds like; all 400 plus attendees eat with the lights off while being served in the dark by blind servers! He highlighted the need that while he was in his political position he had to hide his visual impairment. He now admits that today, he doesn't have to. He further states that although he cannot drive, he holds on to his 20 year old car with the intention that the new breakthroughs in vision research will allow him to once again drive *that* car! I encourage you to read more about them both.

Steve Wynn, the Las Vegas resort and casino developer with retinitis pigmentosa, has kept his condition out of the spotlight, but has been extremely generous in funding research for treatments and cures. I encourage you to find the CBS *60 Minutes* interview with Mr. Wynn that's on YouTube to learn more about this man.

I also must acknowledge Peter Wallsten, the White House correspondent for the *Los Angeles Times,* who has Stargardt's disease. His disease was made a public issue at a White House news briefing when he asked President George W. Bush a question while wearing sunglasses. The President said, "Peter, are you really going to ask me that question wearing those shades?" Peter said, "I can take them off." The President replied, "No, no, leave them on, they look cool. But for the record, it isn't that bright out." And Peter very appropriately responded, "Well, that's a matter of perspective!" Peter reported that the President contacted him later to apologize after being told that Peter was legally blind. I encourage you all to follow Peter's work, as he is incredibly talented.

Then there is young Dr. Tim Cordes, who has Leber's congenital amaurosis and has received his medical degree from the University of Wisconsin. To everyone's astonishment, he has even performed surgery. Dr. Cordes says, "Things are only impossible until they are done!"

Why "Eye Envy"?

Because I only recently identified myself as a sight-impaired person, most of my close friends don't think of me as sight- impaired. Yet one of the toughest challenges and distractions I have is to know I am the only sight-impaired person in many situations. It can make simple interactions with other people awkward.

For instance, unless I'm within two or three feet of people, I can't see their faces. Even at those distances it is quite a struggle. I have been known to walk right past dear friends or family members, unable to recognize them. I understand why it is easy for people to be confused when I tell them that I can't see something and require help. There is always that uncomfortable hesitation. I sit and think about all of those perfect eyes and what I would do if I had better sight. When I see a beautiful sunrise or sunset, and feel the warmth of its beauty, I have to wonder if I will be able to see tomorrow's sun rise or set. There are times when I'm riding my bike, straining to see the road, and someone who I know is a slower cyclist passes me. I always have those little thoughts: "If only I had your eyes." I know this is not a healthy way to think, but these are just thoughts that randomly enter my head. I talk myself through these thoughts, as I do with all my visual challenges. For these reasons, I felt *Eye Envy* was an appropriate title. Envy is rarely healthy, and it's one of the more useless feelings a person can have, especially when there is little that we can do about it.

At the same time, the title *Eye Envy* is a play on words. I know that many of us do the things we do *because* of our disability. I also think it's probable that physically challenged people enjoy a special appreciation of seemingly insignificant accomplishments. By no means am I suggesting that those without some sort of disability don't appreciate their own accomplishments. I am saying that those *with* a disability might have a different perspective on something that another person might not even notice. As I have shared many a race podium with challenged athletes, I know that a lot of us feel more gratitude for just being able to participate in the sport or activity than we do for "winning." Most of the time I am just thrilled to have made it though the day in one piece!

When I started this project, it was to help ease the pain and confusion for newly diagnosed, visually challenged individuals and their families. After the numbing sensation of being diagnosed and now forced to live with such a high degree of uncertainty, most if not all will be filled with fear, loneliness and, quite often, depression. I want to help people cope with this process in a concise, manageable way, while also raising much-needed funds to treat and cure these diseases.

During the process of writing this book, I had the pleasure of meeting hundreds of people, all of whom I found incredibly inspirational, but there was no way I could share each and every story. The support I have from my local community has been amazing. Such people as Yvonne Chester, the Burt family and their son Austin, who has retinitis pigmentosa; Sherri and Carl Kroonenberg with Usher's syndrome; Cheri, Shirley and the rest of the extended Tatem family; and of course Sara Jane and Bill Cohen, have helped me redefine what community means.

All of the people featured in the book generously shared their time and exposed their inner selves to me in an effort to help you and your family understand what you are going through. Most of these people did not themselves have such a resource to help them learn how to cope with their diagnosis and adjust to their new identity. I learned more than words can describe from each of these people, and they took me on an incredible and most unexpected journey. I cannot express enough gratitude.

This is my first book and my first attempt at writing. I worked very hard to maintain the tone and integrity of the conversations I had with those featured. Let their stories inspire you and comfort you, and let the doctors encourage you that help is on the way. Let's just make sure we help *them* help *us*!

Remember: It is not a matter of *whether* treatments or a cure will be found, but *when*.

mls
Boulder, Colorado
June 2010

eye envy

chapter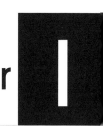

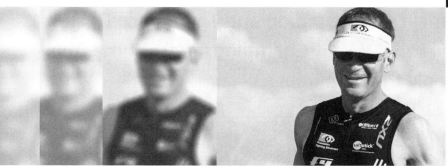

my story

The idea for this book started in the fall of 2006, three years after I was diagnosed with cone-rod dystrophy. So much has changed since then that I am hardly the person I was when I started this project. Today, I am a 10-time Ironman Triathlon finisher. I am also a Regional Champion Xterra Triathlete, earning the Overall Divisional Champion in the Mountain Championship Cup, Third Place Overall Divisional USA Champion and Third Place Overall Divisional World Champion. And I hope this is only the beginning.

I have pursued careers as a hotel/resort developer, philanthropist, personal sports coach and personal trainer. The primary reason I mention these achievements is that I am able to do them despite my disease — I am really not the sort of person to list my accomplishments or give myself accolades. In many ways this disease has taken much, if not all, of my ego.

This chapter is an attempt to let you to get to know me just a little better. We won't be too serious here, as most people who know me will tell you I am rather silly and would rather have those around me smiling and laughing at my life stories, many of which are darn funny.

Due to my efforts noted above, I have received some media attention. Media people ask me, "What inspires you to do the things you do?" It's the question that stumps me the most! I think of the Dr. Seuss book *Oh, The Places You'll Go*, which makes me smile. I think of that little boy and all his adventures that convey one simple truth — that life has many twists and turns.

It has been three years since I started jotting down ideas for this book. I was in such a different emotional place then. As well, I was in such a different place of identity. "Identity" is a word that sums up many thoughts. "Who am I?" is a question I often ask myself, but isn't that something that we all ask ourselves?

Why is it that I should feel any different because I have this vision issue? For some reason I do.

A loss of independence, people treating me differently and daily hardships — all contribute to this feeling. Living with a greater degree of uncertainty affects my day-to-day life. I often wonder, would that have been the case if I had understood my condition years ago? We will never know for me, but we certainly will for those people yet to be diagnosed after these diseases are finally approved for treatment.

My memory of vision-related problems starts when I was about six years old. I am sure my parents have their own memories of this time, but they couldn't see what I was seeing — or wasn't seeing. As I said earlier, I am not blind, but visually challenged. It is a degenerative process and seems to become more challenging each year. I see better in some situations than others, as my visual acuity is based on high contrast. For example, as I write this I am using a computer that has very large white text on a black background. I would prefer yellow text, but I haven't figured out how to make that work. Being computer savvy is not one of my strong suits.

There was a time when I could pass the vision test at the Division of Motor Vehicles. There was a time I could see a baseball moving towards me (although it was difficult). There was a time I could see people's faces, but now I just see people without features unless the conditions are absolutely perfect. At least I *can* see people – although I may not be able to know who I'm talking to, at least I know there's a person there! Most of those featured in this book cannot even see their own faces, much less anyone else's. I can read a book, but require large print and good lighting. Speaking of light, I have now learned that it can be my best friend or worst enemy. Too much light is painful and distorts the image, while not enough light means I see very little of the image. In other words, my vision needs the lighting to be perfect and at the proper angle.

I also have very small blind spots in the center of my vision that make it hard to track moving objects. Watching anything that is backlit is even worse. I have a beautiful 60-inch flat-screen high-definition TV that is very challenging for me to see. I laugh when people see the monster TV in my house and make comments such as, "The neighbors can see that from their house across the street!" But I sit only five feet away from it and *still* struggle to see the images on the screen.

I have difficulty differentiating colors. This became a big problem because a significant aspect of my career involved designing hotels and resorts. At one point, my job included golf course design and development. Prior to my diagnosis, I was working on adding a second golf course at one of our resorts and was working with the golfer Greg Norman. I met with him and his team on several occasions. I knew I couldn't see a golf ball, but I worked hard to keep this a secret during our design talks. I always had an inner laugh to myself and found convenient excuses why I couldn't play golf with the design team.

It has not always been this way, although I am sure my vision was never good. My earliest memories are of seeing large floating shapes that no one else could see. Most of these were in the center of my vision. I would point at the floating shapes to friends and family and they would say they couldn't see them. I thought they were playing a joke on me, which was bizarre and confusing for a six-year-old.

The next memory I have is of my mom being concerned that I would watch TV out of one eye by tilting my head to one side. Apparently it was easier for me to see out of the corner of my peripheral vision.

Throughout my childhood, there were many random but consistent events that indicated I had vision problems. When I was eight, I was playing baseball and was hit in the face with the ball. I recall that what scared me most was that it was a total surprise. I saw the pitcher winding up. I saw the ball leave his hand. And then it smashed into my face. My baseball career was pretty much over after that. To this day I wish I had stuck it out and learned how to compensate for not being able to see the ball fly through the air, but I am not sure how much good that would have done, other than teaching me not to embrace fear, a very important lesson!

Several years later, I went to cheer on a friend at his baseball game. It turned out that not enough players showed up, so the game was forfeited. But since they had the field, both teams agreed to play for fun. They asked me to participate, to round out the numbers. Since I couldn't see the ball and was stuck in right field, I watched which direction the infielders were looking to figure out if the ball was headed my way. One problem with that plan: I still couldn't figure out which way to run to catch the ball. I had no idea the other kids could see things I couldn't. I just remember the angry complaints: "F**k, he's running the wrong way. He sucks!!!" That has haunted me ever since.

Unfortunately this affected my entire view of sports in general. I became one of the last picked in P.E. I found every excuse to get myself out of team sports. Even the idea of individual sports, such as running, was too intimidating. I used every excuse I could find to avoid participating.

Back then, if someone had predicted that one day I would race an Ironman, which consists of swimming 2.4 miles, biking 112 miles and then running 26.2 miles (all of which must be done consecutively in under 17 hours), I would have laughed that person off. And if he'd then told me that I would do this multiple times in my life and earn trophies for it, I'd have had some serious doubts about his sanity!

The next challenges came with music, for which I always have had a passion. I started playing piano at a very young age, and then the trombone, flute, tuba and guitar. Learning instruments came easily to me. As time went by, though, sight-reading music became more difficult. In hindsight, I realize it was the brightness of the page that washed out the notes on the page, as opposed to the music notes being too small. I started to memorize my parts and simply play from memory. No one told me to do this; it was just something I figured out on my own. To this day that's what I do. Although I have a strong ear for music, reading music is impossible unless I take the score to a photocopy store and enlarge the print. This slightly improves the contrast and gives me a fighting chance to see the notes. It is still very difficult, as it doesn't fix the contrast problem and I am still using the same memorizing technique I did as a young musician. The problem was that because no one seemed to notice that I had trouble reading music, I got by.

Of course, if I couldn't see a page of musical notes that was within a foot of me, how could I see a chalkboard or a projector screen? As obvious as it might seem, we don't know what we don't see. If a child can't communicate what he doesn't see, and doesn't know that he isn't seeing an image, how can he effectively participate in his education?

Teachers are not responsible for diagnosing

vision problems. They assume that each child is tested, and that kids who have vision problems are prescribed eyeglasses. However, the schools' vision tests, much like the DMV's, don't use sophisticated equipment. They certainly don't test for visual field or contrast. Ophthalmologists have equipment that can do so, but it was not used to test me until much later in life. When I was a kid, an optometrist could correct my vision to be somewhat adequate, but I was unable to explain the other problems I was having because I was unaware that I was "missing" anything.

If a child isn't paying attention or is doodling, teachers naturally become frustrated. Mine certainly did! Not getting my homework completed was my worst problem. I was way too young to think to ask what the assignments were if I couldn't see them written on the chalkboard. Some teachers were better than others, but most didn't hesitate to tell me they had little sympathy for a student who was a nuisance. Of course, my homework took hours for me to read over, do, and review. Few kids have the ability to focus for such a long period of time, and I was no exception.

Unfortunately, this pattern continued throughout high school and into my early university days. It took me a while to realize that I performed better when teachers did not use sight-based teaching aids such as chalkboards or overhead projectors. High school was particularly challenging because almost all teachers used "visual aids" to instruct. At the end of my sophomore year I pleaded with my parents to find me some help – but not for my vision, as I still didn't understand what it was I didn't see. A business partner of my father's mentioned boarding school as a good option, and my parents helped make this reality. Of course, there are some negative associations with sending a teenager to boarding school in the middle of his high school years. As soon as I went off to the school we found in northern Massachusetts, the rumor mill started up: "Did you hear Michael Stone was sent away? I heard it was drugs … !"

I assure anyone reading this that drugs were never part of my life, and anyone who knows me well would laugh at that thought. Even today my friends have to coax me to have a glass of wine. Luckily my parents never gave me much reason to rebel. I had my share of hobbies, and they supported each of them. I even had a snake collection. How many moms would allow that?

I was 16 when I went to boarding school, where I did well academically. In fact at one point I ranked fourth in my class. This was a far cry from my low ranking at public school. I often asked myself why my performance had improved. The workload was greater than in public school and equally challenging, if not more so. But most of the classes only had 10 or so students, and the chalkboard was only a few feet away. We sat at conference-room tables rather than desks. The classrooms that did have desks were a greater challenge, but I still managed to get through those classes since the classrooms were very small. It never occurred to any of us that my sight was the culprit.

That year, however, I *did* start to notice how sensitive my vision was to light. I played on the soccer team, and my ophthalmologist gave me a pair of prescription sunglasses. They didn't look very good, but they certainly helped. After one year at private school I went back to finish public school with my friends, hoping that my success in private school would carry over. Well, not exactly. I made it through and graduated, but it wasn't pretty.

By the time I was in university, the professors in my majors didn't use as many visual aids and simply lectured. But I still struggled academically while at the University of Miami. I still didn't know what my visual problem was.

In 1991 I began working as a real estate investment analyst/asset manager in Chicago. Most of my work was done on a computer. Computers were certainly not what they are today. But by the mid-1990s we were using laptop computers more than the desktop PCs. It was easier for me to get closer to the laptop screen due to its portability. The images on the computer screen had become increasingly difficult for me to see, and my colleagues were horrified by how close I got to the screen. They couldn't figure out why I preferred a small-screen laptop as opposed to a large-screen PC. The truth was I couldn't see any better with a desktop monitor. It never occurred to me or anyone else that the lack of contrast was the problem. I started to dim the brightness as much as possible, but it was little help.

In 1993, I discovered rock climbing. This was the start of many amazing adventures. My climbing friends and I made weekend excursions to various "crags" around the country. We camped out and arose early to climb sheer rock faces. Many of these climbs were what is called "sport climbing." We clipped carabiners (spring hooks attached to webbing and a rope) into bolts attached to the rock face and then climbed the route using the rope and hand and foot holds, which are small shapes or cracks in the rock.

The bolts showed us the route we were meant to take. Most of these climbs had some 10 bolts to the top. I was lucky if I could see the first bolt, while my friends would see all the way to the top of the route. Once again, contrast was the key. How could I see a little silver bolt that was intentionally designed to blend into the rock face? I couldn't, but I still managed to lead my way up these climbs. I climbed some of America's most famous routes, but seeing the tiny hand and foot holds on the rock surface became more challenging as my vision changed. I began to find hand and foot holds by feel. This meant a very long day for my partners and me, as the climbs took several times longer than they used to. It meant doing a single climb in a day, as opposed to several climbs. I was fortunate to have very patient and supportive friends.

In August of 1997, I moved to Boulder, Colorado. I wanted a change from Chicago and I very much loved rock climbing. I learned to climb traditional routes, which is a different technique from sport climbing. Instead of attaching to permanent bolts in the rock face, you use temporary devices that are taken out either when you descend, or by a follower on her way up. This also had challenges, but I didn't need to see the bolts anymore.

Of course it did mean that I needed to see the route well enough to know what protection to bring if I was going to lead. I just brought everything I might possibly need with me! I'm sure I was an amusing sight overloaded with all that gear.

In 2000, my Chicago climbing friends came out to Boulder for a seasonal climbing trip. Some of us signed up for Boulder's renowned 10-kilometer running race, the Bolder Boulder. Although I had never run three miles, much less six, I figured, "Oh well, why not?!" I must say finishing in the stadium with thousands of cheering people was one of the greatest feelings of my life. My race was not fast or pretty, and I knew nothing about running technique or endurance. But I could climb and hike, and that made the transition from rock climbing to running a little easier.

At that time, I was also doing a little road biking. When I moved to Boulder, the only person I knew was a work colleague who told me, "If you live in Boulder, you need a road bike." And so it was. I bought a bike knowing little to nothing of what I was buying. In fact, I had no idea how to shift the brake lever shifters! I brought the bike back to the bike shop after my first ride around my apartment's parking lot and told the mechanic, "The shifters will only shift in one direction." The nice mechanic put it on the stand and shifted through each and every gear perfectly. I walked out red faced.

So, I was cycling a little and periodically running. I found myself a series of personal trainers who tried to turn me into a power weight lifter. I would work out early in the morning with these trainers. Every morning during my training sessions people came to the weight room with soaking-wet hair to hop on a spinning bike or a treadmill. I couldn't figure out why they showered before their workout! Finally, I asked a nice woman why this was. She looked at me as if I was crazy and told me she had just finished swimming in a master's class.

The athletes would swim their master's class for about 90 minutes and then rode a bike or ran for another hour or more. Needless to say, I thought this was amazing. "Why so much?" I asked her. She said she was training for a triathlon. I found my heart pumping with both excitement and envy. She seemed so happy and was filled with pride. Yes, this was definitely for me!

I ran my second Bolder Boulder in May 2001, 10 minutes faster than the previous year's time. Again, not so pretty, but it still felt amazing. I took a few swim lessons and decided to try a triathlon. I had no idea what training meant. I figured, "You swim a little, bike a little and run a little and you'll be fine." I had much to learn.

It turned out that the woman who helped me with my swimming was Missy Arthur, a prominent Boulder triathlete and personal trainer.

She signed me up for my inaugural race, the Loveland Lake to Lake Triathlon, held in Loveland, Colorado. It took place one month after my second Bolder Boulder, in June of 2001.

Generally in life I try to be prepared, like a good Boy Scout! I bought all the gear Missy said I would need, such as a wetsuit and something to wear for all three events. Generally for a race of this distance, you wear one piece of clothing for all three events. But there was so much I didn't know. Where should I put all of my stuff? How would I transition from one event to another? What should I eat and drink? The night before the race, I was all registered, but was panicking at the realization that I had no clue what I had gotten myself into. I asked my friend Kam Zardouzian, a two-time Ironman triathlete, what I was supposed to do. He explained the transition area to me and gave me a video of a professional race. The video featured a professional triathlete, Wes Hobson, and several others as they raced in a national championship event in Southern California. These men and women ran, swam and biked so fast that I felt absolutely zero confidence in what I was about to do early the next morning. Wes and I coincidentally became very close friends, and I will discuss more about my friendship with him and his family in another section.

On race morning, the forecast was for temperatures of over 100 degrees. I had heard on NPR that during the week before the race there had been an *E. coli* outbreak in Loveland Lake, but I just told myself I wouldn't allow any water in my mouth. Anyone who has seen or experienced a triathlon swim knows how ridiculous the notion of "not allowing water in your mouth" really is.

The race started very late. As forecast, the temperatures rose past 100. In a wetsuit that was at least two sizes too large, I was sweating out what little fluid I had in my body. When the starter horn went off, we all began swimming at a pace ridiculously faster than I had ever practiced during my three or four training swims. I kept bumping into other swimmers and stopping to apologize. The others looked at me as if I was crazy. I thought their assessment was fair, as I had no business being there. Approximately 200 yards into the 1500-meter swim I swallowed a mouthful of water and promptly gagged, thinking about the *E. coli* outbreak that only I seemed to know about. The swim course followed a line of buoys directly into the sun. I couldn't see any of them. Well, I wasn't the last person out of the water, but was fairly close to that.

Then it was time for the bike ride. I heard a man getting on his bike apologize to his wife for taking so long in the swim. Since I was right there with him, I knew I must be near the back of the herd. But of the three triathlon disciplines, I was best at cycling. Although once again I found seeing the course a challenge, I still didn't know it was different for me than for anyone else. I started passing other competitors with relative ease. I played a game in my head that day as I passed yet another athlete. I called each one "Herman." I don't know why that name popped into my head, but it made the time go by faster and it was fun, albeit secretly obnoxious! I would say under my breath, "Nice riding, Herman. See you on the run." Luckily none of them heard me say it — or if they did, they ignored me. I later found out that a sports psychologist friend of mine now uses this story with his clients, calling it "picking off the Hermans."

As I finished the bike portion and headed out for the run I found it very confusing, as there were people everywhere. Approximately a mile and a half into the run I ran past a directional person who said, "This way!" Somehow I missed the directional signs — I never saw any of them. I headed off in the direction she indicated, only to find myself 12 minutes later at the finish line, hearing congratulatory cheers.

"Uh, I think there was a mistake … I don't run a 24-minute 10K!" I realized I'd only run three miles instead of six, so I headed back toward where I'd begun. By the time I crossed the finish line *again*, I had run nine miles instead of six. Since I was barely prepared to run six miles, much less nine, I finished my first triathlon with very little fuel left. But I was now a triathlete! I had no idea where this new identity would take me.

Triathlon has several different distances. Quite often people confuse the word "triathlon" with Ironman. I am frequently asked, "Do you do the full triathlon?" All triathlons consist of swimming, biking and running, in that sequence. The only difference is the distance you do. The shortest distances are called sprints, and they increase to Olympic or international, then Half Ironman (now called 70.3 for the total distance in miles), then Ironman. Both 70.3 and Ironman are registered trademarks of the World Triathlon Corporation (WTC). There is even an Ultraman that has its own incredibly long distance.

I wasn't really fast enough to fully enjoy and appreciate the shorter Olympic distance courses. They generally consist of a 1500-meter swim, followed by a bike stage that is usually about

40 kilometers, topped off by a 10-kilometer run. I raced one more of these and then decided that I should try a longer course. I tend to not do anything the "easy way," so I chose to race a Half Ironman in Pucón, Chile, in February of 2002. This time I determined I would train properly. I asked Kathleen Motylenski, an experienced personal trainer at my local gym, to help me train for Chile. I was unaware of what coaches do and was truly clueless about what to do next. I had never completed any of the distances of a Half Ironman (a 1.2-mile swim, 56-mile bike, followed by a 13.1-mile run). This time I trained for three months and through the winter. I did everything I was told to. Kathleen was very clever about how she held me back and kept my effort slow and steady. It worked just fine. Still, I had no idea what to expect, as I was very intimidated by the distances.

Standing at the start for the Half Ironman, I once again felt out of my league when I saw the other athletes. They were built like machines, ready to handle anything thrown at them. I was most certainly not. But it didn't matter! I came in under the seven-hour cutoff for the race, while several others did not. The race was incredibly challenging, but so beautiful. At the finish line I broke down in tears. It was the most amazing experience in my life up to that point.

After finishing, I thought about all of those teachers who had belittled me while I was growing up. I thought about being one of the last people picked for teams in P.E. class. Finishing the Half Ironman was harder than any mountain I had climbed, but well worth the effort. And yet I thought, "There is no way I would ever race a full Ironman. This was challenging enough!"

However, a year later almost to the day, I completed my first full Ironman in New Zealand. It's hard for me to believe that I have since completed 10 full Ironman races, 25 Half Ironman races, scores of running, swimming and cycling events, and many triathlons. The tally of these races will increase, as I have no intention of stopping. I also have become a certified triathlon coach and personal trainer and helped many others achieve such goals.

Yet, despite all these accomplishments, I felt that I was not achieving my athletic potential. There was always some impediment to my progress as a triathlete. The swim portion was always a struggle to sight the buoys. The bike portion had its own challenges with obstacles in the road, and the run — well, that was just plain hard. I would miss curbs here and there and sometimes step in holes. When I ran off-road on trails, I kept turning my ankles by stepping on rocks and roots. I just couldn't run with confidence or train at my best. I didn't know that this wasn't normal.

In 2003, during the bike portion of the New Zealand Ironman, I rode right past the person who held a directional sign that signaled a very important turn. Normally the sign holders yell out in advance when racers are approaching an important turn. However, this time no one called out to warn me, and with no riders in front to lead the way and being unable to see the sign, I missed the turn. Missing that turn was very upsetting, to say the least. That, plus the combination of feeling that I was underachieving athletically and being denied my driver's license at the DMV, finally pushed me to figure out what was causing my problems.

My ophthalmogist in Chicago, Dr. Coleman Kraff, worked hard at trying to diagnose what was going on with my sight. But after many appointments, a brain MRI and an attempt at Lasik surgery, Dr. Kraff advised me to consult with an expert in neuro-ophthalmology. He referred me to his colleague and former professor at the University of Illinois, Dr. James Goodwin.

Most of the experts I have consulted over the years theorized that I had strained optic nerves, which was why my vision couldn't be corrected. But after a battery of tests, Dr. Goodwin found nothing wrong with my optic nerves. However, he did see a few blind spots in my central vision. He walked me down the hall

to visit one of his colleagues, Dr. Gerald Fishman, a famous retina specialist. We found Dr.
Fishman eating lunch at his desk, but he graciously agreed to give me a quick exam in his
tiny office.

To conduct the exam, Dr. Fishman used a
common technique of retinoscopy to look at
the back of my eye. While he did so, other
doctors talked away about what they what
they thought I had, as if I were not even in the
room. They said horrifying things about my
central "blind spots." The more they talked,
the more anxious I became. Dr. Fishman took
a break from his exam and said, "Don't you
just love when people are talking about you
right in front of you, as if you were not in the
room?" I knew I had the right guy!

After another few minutes, he took a deep
breath and then asked me rhetorical questions that described my life experiences, although I hadn't told him any of my symptoms.
I was 36 years old and had struggled most of
my life without being able to describe how I

saw — or how I didn't see — and finally had a doctor who understood what was going on. "Well, I know what you have and you will have a long road ahead," Dr. Fishman told me. I really didn't want to ask what that meant. I desperately tried to hold back the fear and sadness that welled up in me.

Dr. Fishman was amazed that I had been able to get through school without help. He was saddened that it took so long for me to be diagnosed. The truth is I always felt that there was more going on about my vision than I was told. When I was a child, *Little House on the Prairie* was a popular show. I remember the scene where one of the children lost her sight due to scarlet fever. I was horrified by that scene and had nightmares about it throughout my life. I always felt a connection. In fact, just after I had Lasik surgery and was able to see fairly well for the first time in my life, I told an ophthalmogist friend of mine, "I hope it holds." He said, "Michael, this is your vision!" And although I hoped he was correct, I never really believed him.

Dr. Fishman said I had a disease called cone-rod dystrophy, an inherited retinal degenerative disease. Although he felt sure his diagnosis was correct, he needed to run some tests to confirm his assessment. The first test was an electroretinogram, or ERG. This eye test detects abnormal function in the retina, the light-detecting portion of the eye. The light-sensitive cells (rods and cone cells) in the retina are examined. During the test, an electrode is placed on the cornea (at the front of the eye) that measures how well the cells in the back of the eye (the retina) sense light.

To do this test, my eyes were dilated and my lids were propped open. It was uncomfortable and frightening. I was put in a dark room where I waited for about 20 minutes for my eyes to adjust to the darkness. As soon as my eyes adjusted to the darkness, bright lights that seemed like strobe lights were flashed directly into my eyes. Because I am light sensitive, this was close to torture for me. The test itself took about 20 minutes. It confirmed Dr. Fishman's diagnosis.

I felt numb but at the same time overwhelmed with emotion. How did this man diagnose what no one else could, with only a simple silver-dollar-size lens? Why did it take so many years to confirm what I had always felt and feared? Yet the diagnosis made sense. It explained all those years of struggle with my schoolteachers. It explained the aggravation I caused my brothers and parents by constantly displacing my frustration onto them.

After the exam my eyes were so dilated that I could barely see well enough to get back to my parents' home. Here I was, just diagnosed with a blindness-related disease, and the tests for diagnosing my illness caused me temporarily to have worse sight than ever before. I didn't really understand my diagnosis well enough to explain it to anyone.

In an effort to flag down a taxi, I waved at every yellow car that I detected. It took a long while before a taxi stopped, and then I couldn't see the meter. (I still can't). Although I knew my vision would be restored to its "normal" state in a day or so, I couldn't help but think about all the people who experienced this every day, and the trust they must have just to get through life's most basic requirements. I felt extremely alone. It's a feeling that no one should ever have to experience.

Back in Boulder, I was in denial mode for months. At the time of the diagnosis I didn't ask many questions, not even whether there were treatments or cures. Eventually, I started doing a little Web research. I searched for cone-rod dystrophy but there wasn't much information available. I found a couple of pages of holistic companies that believed they had natural remedies for this and other eye-related problems. I found a couple of pages written by others with cone-rod dystrophy. What I read horrified me: One man was learning Braille; another was learning to work with a seeing-eye dog. My stomach lurched with fear.

Something else I learned was that not only was *I* in denial, but so were my parents. Although I had told them about Dr. Fishman's diagnosis, I kept it brief and simple. I really didn't know what I was talking about, anyway. I realized it was time for me to be more proactive about my situation. Just over one year after my diagnosis, my mom mentioned the situation to a friend of hers, who suggested I talk to Sue Abnerholden, who formerly worked for the Foundation Fighting Blindness (FFB). Sue was very friendly and sent me heaps of information. I told Sue that I would like to dedicate my next Ironman race to the Foundation Fighting Blindness. I was familiar with degenerative genetic diseases, as I had been racing to benefit cystic fibrosis research. I have a very special friend in New Zealand with this dreadful disease. Her name is Kimberley Robottom and she and her family are special people who have supported me beyond words. I use fundraising for charities as a motivator, and it has evolved into my having a second family.

As we had already received conflicting information about my own "problem" (I wasn't calling it a disease yet), my dad felt it was time to talk to Dr. Fishman directly and I made a trip that winter to Chicago. Dr. Fishman explained how the "problem" would affect my range of vision. He could not say exactly what my process would be, however, and made a profound comment about living with uncertainty. He shared with us his own struggles with heart problems. And he explained the genetic statistics — something my friend Dr. Joanna Zeiger, a world champion triathlete and epidemiologist, would have to explain several times over to me.

I decided to race Ironman Wisconsin for FFB in September 2005. I created a Web site and used a charity I founded that encourages athletes to race for charities they choose. Sue helped me write the Web page and I started my first fundraiser for FFB. This was a strange sensation that felt a little self-serving, but it was the only way I could feel proactive and not just idly wait for the deepening vision loss that Dr. Fishman predicted for me.

The race was tough, in conditions harsher than I had ever experienced. We triathletes like to think that our most recent race is *always* the toughest race, but this one truly was! Even though it was my fifth Ironman, it was the first race that my family watched. It was also interesting that it had taken me so long to become proactive in the fight against blindness. My grandfather had passed away only a couple of months prior to this race. He finished his life suffering from macular degeneration. Although it started to affect him later in life, I am sad to admit how long it took my family and me to acknowledge his battle. This didn't occur to me until Sue introduced me to a brother and sister, both with Usher's syndrome, who were supporting the race. It felt as if this was my first time in the presence of people with degenerative eye diseases, but it clearly was not. To this day I feel ashamed that I didn't become active in the fight against blindness before I was diagnosed with cone-rod dystrophy.

The Wisconsin weather was extremely hot, hitting temperatures in the mid-90s, accompanied by powerful winds. And then something happened at the beginning of the bike portion that had never happened before: I crashed! A couple of athletes in front of me hadn't secured their water bottles properly, and the bottles were jettisoned after the riders hit a major bump in the road. One of the bottles lodged in my front wheel, which sent me over the handlebars, smashing to the ground. There I was on the roadside, only an hour and a half into the day and only one kilometer into the 180-kilometer bike portion. My handlebars and front wheel were broken, my shoulder was badly injured, I was a bloody mess, and my nutrition for the race was spilled on the ground. But my parents and brothers were waiting for me somewhere along the course – there was no way this was going to be the end of my day! For over 20 minutes I lay on the ground, trying to make a plan. Finally I picked myself up and started pedaling my barely rideable bike. My mind was not as much in the race as thinking of all who supported me. Part of me felt embarrassment, but I also felt motivated more than ever to hit that finish line! I rode most of the bike portion with one arm. It was way too painful for me to try to grip with both hands, and my arm didn't want to properly bend. I was denied medical attention at the second transition, because the medical staff were overwhelmed by the numbers of people who needed help, due to either dehydration or hyponatremia (basically an extreme loss of sodium in the blood). The medical staff told me I would have to pull out of the race if I were to receive medical aid. Clearly that wasn't an option, so off on the run I went!

I ran the marathon holding my arm steady with my other hand, as my shoulder was badly swollen. It wasn't long until I saw my dad at the side of the road trying to run alongside in an effort to take my photo. This was all the motivation I needed. There is no better feeling than having a loved one excited to see you race. I finished the race with both my brothers running the finish line arm-in-arm with me. It was a magical moment that I will never forget. It was my hardest and best effort, and it was amazing! The funny thing is I made my best placement ever, because so many athletes pulled out of the race.

The only part that was hard to swallow was: Why was I the only one to crash there? I really didn't want to think it had anything to do with my vision, but I know the crash might have been avoided if I could better see such ob-stacles. I know that fully sighted people crash, but this felt unique.

A Change of Identity

My fundraising effort at Ironman Wisconsin signaled the start of a new life for me.

After the Wisconsin race, the Foundation Fighting Blindness made me their cover story for their annual report. For this story, I was interviewed by the Foundation's public rela-tions director, Allie Laban-Baker. I had never really been interviewed before. I figured I'd be asked about racing Ironmans and fundraising, but I couldn't have been more wrong. Allie caught me off guard by asking me about my childhood experiences coping with having vision loss, and my relationship with my teachers. Reality hit me, hard. In fact, I was deeply depressed for several weeks after that interview.

But Allie also did me a great favor: For the first time, I turned to my friends to help me through my depression. They really helped me focus on getting "healthy" and advised me to leave some of my commitments for another day. I will never forget the advice my friend Joanna gave me that bad week: "Your health is far more important than anything else. Everything else can wait for you." She was right! Sadly, this meant having to give up the puppy I had taken in just that week — not an easy thing to do for a dog lover. Joanna and her husband, Mark, went with me to deliver the puppy to his new home.

The Foundation's article resulted in my raising funds for them *again* by participating in the 2006 Ironman World Championship. This opportunity came about through Dr. Kraff, the Chicago ophthalmologist who referred me to Dr. Fishman. Dr. Kraff and his father shared the Foundation's feature about me with Dr. James Gills, then-owner of Ironman and a cornea expert. Dr. Gills contacted me and invited me to race that year at the World Championship in Kona, Hawaii. It was a dream come true. I promised that I would make the very most of this gift by raising more funds for retinal research.

FFB made me a dedicated page on their Web site. The media began contacting me. I received hundreds of emails from strangers who wanted to share their own stories as well as ask me questions. I made several television appearances and was featured in newspaper articles and magazines. It was a fascinating experience and only the beginning of much more to come. I can do fundraiser after fundraiser, but if the collective "we" are ever going to maximize our potential for raising funds, we have to have more people racing for this cause. For example, a triathlete named Sally Mitchell, living in New York, formed a group of fully sighted athletes to race the New York City Triathlon for our cause. I had the pleasure of coaching them through that race.

A few weeks before the World Championship Ironman, my youngest brother, Russell, called to tell me of some recent challenges he was having. It sounded way too familiar to me. He asked if he should make an appointment with Dr. Fishman. I said he should, but he should not go alone! As it turned out, he too has cone-rod dystrophy. I can't express how bad I felt when he was diagnosed. Luckily, at this writing my brother has not had the same challenges I have, but he is also six years younger. Still, it added an element that I was no longer alone in the battle. It helped me further understand how these diseases are inherited.

And then, soon after Russell's diagnosis, I raced in the Ironman World Championship in Hawaii. Bad luck seemed to be dogging me. First, my brother's diagnosis and second, I had a femoral injury. Third, an earthquake hit Hawaii that week. And fourth, heavy rains falling throughout the day soaked much of the racecourse. My poor parents waited 12 hours, standing in waist-deep water, for me to reach the finish line! The aspect I love most about racing Ironman and triathlon in general is that it is inherently understood that there will be down moments as well as up moments. We need to prepare for both. All it takes is one good moment to forget all the bad moments. I find racing to be a metaphor for life, and that is probably why I enjoy racing so much. Racing in Hawaii was by far not my greatest race, but it's a race that's beyond special in my heart and memory. Having my parents there was incredible. Having my family and friends' support, and the support of my new community of visually impaired athletes and their families, is what really made the experience wonderful.

The Hawaii Ironman fundraising went very well. My parents held fundraisers in Florida and Chicago, one for each group of friends.

Our collective effort raised over $250,000 and much more since.

The media attention was frightening and exciting. The fright was caused by some of the media portraying me as being already blind. I still hadn't accepted that I was going blind, and didn't even know what being blind would mean for me. The excitement was from an article in *Triathlete Magazine* about the Hawaii Ironman that mentioned the overall champions, past champions *and me* all in one sentence. Several friends told me about the article. In many ways, that was the most rewarding media attention I received, being included in an article about champions.

The amazing people I met at Ironman Hawaii hold a special place in my heart, and I remain in contact with many of them. A few are featured in this book. Also, as a result of the pre- and post-race publicity, I received hundreds of calls and emails from other individuals and families affected by retinal disease. I met several other visually challenged athletes who did their best to share their experiences with me. They have become friends from afar and have helped me with racing with the challenges we face. Two of these people require special mention as they continue to race despite their vision challenges. They are Ryan Van Praet and Maverick Malech, both very talented athletes. Several other young people I met through this experience have made all the hard work that much more rewarding. Nick Kalyan and Zach Chadwick, both teenagers with retinitis pigmentosa, really helped push me to work harder and to be a better athlete and person. I know I have to make my way back to Ironman Hawaii some day, but right now there are just so many other races that I am enjoying!

There are three categories of athletes in these races: professionals, age groupers (subdivided into groups by age) and physically challenged. Physically challenged athletes are also subdivided into groups based on their specific challenge: wheelchair, amputee or visually challenged. To this day I choose to race road

triathlons without the title of "physically challenged," as I still have significant sight that allows me to race as an individual age grouper
and wish to hold onto that status as long as
they will allow me. The rules in these races dic-
tate that we be spaced out both for safety and
so we don't have an advantage from "draft-
ing" from a cyclist in front of us. Of course it is
challenging for me, and sometimes scary, but
as long as I feel it merely slows me a little and
is not a safety issue for my fellow competitors,
I will keep racing as I am.

Back to Today

I feel that there are two Michaels — the old
me, and the new one. Although the new me
sometimes lives in the shadow of the old me,
the new me has been liberated by the explanation for his vision struggles. The old me went
through life as best he could, but with much
anger and frustration that the challenges he
faced had no answer. The new me is very
much aware of the problems I face due to my

deteriorating vision, but is focused on making the most of each day, and is reconstructing his life.

This is the work in progress I spoke of. How one begins to reconstruct one's life is probably something for psychologists to determine. I know they have identified stages that we have to go through, such as grieving, anger, acceptance, etc. I'm sure I'm butchering the list, but my point is that these stages are personal and unique to each individual. I don't believe that any two people share the same experience. My experience has been more of a revolution of all the stages as I have gone through them out of order. The one I have not really experienced is "acceptance." What am I supposed to accept? Acceptance dictates that I will have to live with a degree of uncertainty that I will eventually lose more sight over an unspecified amount of time without knowing precisely how much sight will be lost. I suppose I can acknowledge it and move on, but with each day bringing different developments in my sightedness, what I'm accepting constantly changes. Perhaps acceptance is about being comfortable with being uncomfortable. Everyone has to live with some uncertainty. They might choose to ignore this fact, but nevertheless it is there. The difference is that people with RDDs still have *that* uncertainty plus the added one that comes with our disease.

When I embarked on the exercise of writing this book, it was to answer these questions I asked of myself: How can I do everything in my power to help those affected and their families cope with these diseases after their diagnosis? How can I do all that I can to raise funds to find treatments and cures?

The doctors can only do so much when they give us a diagnosis. They are not responsible for comforting us afterwards. This might seem obvious, but I have seen much anger targeted at the people delivering the bad news. Providing and finding comfort is our responsibility and the responsibility of our loved ones. I had to ask myself, "Is there anything I can possibly do to fill in the blanks?" Well, the answer to this remains unclear. I will say that through the amorphous evolution that led me to this book, there has been enormous change — dare I say growth — in my own life. One important detail is that I most certainly do not feel as alone. I used to feel as if I was the only person in the world who had this specific vision problem. But now when I'm in a space with a thousand people, I wonder who else has this problem or something similar.

An important realization I had while interviewing people for this book is that after my diagnosis, I had become exactly what I was trying to avoid: fearful. I had become filled with fear — fear of leaving the house, fear of trying new things, fear of living outside my comfort zone. You might wonder what is outside the comfort zone of someone who's completed 10 Ironman races in six years. Racing an Ironman is well within my comfort zone. Indeed, it's too much in my comfort zone. Spending my time swimming, biking and running is very comfortable for me. However, what *is* outside my comfort zone is sharing my vision loss with those closest to me.

During the period when I was trying to understand what my diagnosis meant, and how to confront my fears about its effect on my life, I was also in a romantic relationship. I wasn't looking for sympathy, but I did need emotional support, some physical assistance, and time to understand what was going on — I needed my partner to help me. I couldn't seem to show my partner that my vision issues caused me to live in constant fear. She would quite often tell me "This has nothing to do with vision" when I was showing reluctance to do something that she wanted. But living in fear affected everything I did, right down to blinking and sleeping, as I said above.

The emotional effects were pervasive. For example, in many large gatherings I cannot identify faces and frequently am disoriented, especially at outdoor venues where the light can be too bright for me to see much more than glare and movement. During that time of adjustment, I sometimes felt frozen with fear in social situations. Therefore, I asked my partner to stay close by and tell me who was at the event or approaching me. Although I did my best to share how difficult this was for me, she didn't or couldn't understand what I was going through. She was unable to wait out this period of adjustment and adjust to my changing needs. I truly did not understand the changes I was going through or how hard it was to face the fear that was weighing in on me. Not be able to share with her the true extent of my vision loss and how it affected me, coupled with her lack of willingness or capability to understand, cost me that relationship.

I learned much from that experience, as sad as it was. We need to understand *what* it is we need help with, and *how* to ask people to help us. We have to communicate directly to our friends, family and lovers. In turn, they need to be honest and let us know what they can or cannot do. Can they deal with our physical disability? Are they able to cope with our specific needs that are different from the sighted community's? I still have concerns and fear about whether friends and family will be here for me when I need them, even after having honest conversations about my disease and how it may affect me. They have their own lives to live and I know they will always do their best to help me when they can. I am especially anxious because my sight continues to degenerate daily and I know that what I don't need help with today may be something I do need help with tomorrow, or next week or next month. And that's difficult to explain or share with someone who doesn't have a progressive disability.

I realize now that over the past few years, I have found it more and more difficult to break out of my routines and safe haven. Some days, just leaving my home was difficult. This is generally due to emotional exhaustion from dealing with changes I am experiencing from greater vision loss. Of course, there is little safety in *not* making the most of your day. There is only regret. At the same time, breaking a routine is a constant challenge.

However, there's always something for me to do to occupy my brain or satisfy my thirst for adventure. More to the point, I want to minimize my sense of regret that I didn't make the most of the vision I have at any moment, even if it is changing day by day.

By no means have I figured this out. I envy the people who have. Many of those featured in this book have found their niche in life and continue to make the most of every day. I know each of them has up and down moments, as do people who don't have RDDs. The biggest difference is that we have the usual up and down moments, plus the ups and downs that disease adds to the mix. I often hear people who don't have a physical disability try to diminish their own personal experience with loss or a bad day by suggesting, "Well, my experience is nothing like yours." I feel bad that they feel they need to do this. A bad day is a bad day. Of course it could be worse! We can make ourselves crazy with that kind of thought process. The best we can all do is play the cards we are dealt the best we can. We just need to go one step further and allow ourselves the luxury of having a bad moment, and we can always gain more tools to move through these bad moments.

As I set out to write a book that would educate and inspire those directly affected with vision loss (those who have RDDs and their close friends and family members), I never thought that *I* needed this emotional catharsis! I learned so much from the people featured in this book, and I hold their stories close to me. I frequently receive letters from them about their progress and am so thankful that they have the courage to share their stories with me and you. They represent an enormous group of ordinary people who do extraordinary things. Their stories inspired me to see myself for who I had become and taught me that I could choose to move beyond fear.

Being Comfortable with Being Uncomfortable and Finding Limitations

For me, the year 2009 was a test to find my

own limitations, inspired by the people I had interviewed for this book. The test began with a return to skiing (actually, learning skate-skiing), then returning to trail running and taking on mountain biking. As I said, racing in an Ironman was well within my comfort zone, but I had been envious of those who could race off road; it was something I *knew* I just couldn't do. I couldn't even run the trails behind my house anymore, as I constantly sprained my ankles on rocks and other obstacles that I couldn't see. I frequently fell flat on my face, bruised my ribs and left much skin on those trails. My envy was fed by my then-girlfriend, who almost exclusively participated in off-road running races and would return home saying, "You would have hated this, it would have been too hard for you." She might have been trying to relate to me, but all it did was dig a deeper hole in my heart, as I wanted to be out there with her. The same held true for skiing, which I gave up even before my diagnosis. For some reason, I kept crashing while skiing. I had skied my entire life without problems, and all of a sudden I had bad crashes and more close calls than I cared to admit. So I had given up two sports that I loved.

I was surprised when my friend Jamie Whitmore, who was coping with her own woes fighting cancer, suggested I try racing an off-road triathlon called Xterra. Jamie was an Xterra World Champion, and she knew of another visually challenged athlete who raced off-road with a guide. The guide helped the athlete with swimming, cycling and running by calling out commands. This of course piqued my interest, but filled me with fear and excitement. I love to try new things and hate the idea that there is anything I cannot be or do just because I don't see well. However, the Xterra triathlon was no easy feat for me, especially learning how to ride a mountain bike.

My first experience on a mountain bike was devastating. After purchasing my bike I waited for my friends, who said they would ride with me, to take me on the trails. After waiting some time, I decided to head out alone just for 20 minutes on the flat portion of the trails behind my house. It was definitely safe enough. I knew these trails very well, having lived on them for eight years. They are essentially off-road walking paths with almost no obstacles aside from the huge community of prairie dogs and the occasional rattlesnake.

I did OK going out, but had problems with the return trip home. Approximately 30 seconds along a trail I thought would take me home, I realized I was going in the wrong direction, and promptly turned around. When I hit the bottom of the trail, there was a furious runner awaiting me. He yelled at me, "This trail is off limits to bikes!" I said, "I am so sorry, I was lost." He responded, "Are you f***ing blind? There's a sign right there!"

I looked over to where he was pointing and couldn't see a sign. I moved closer and closer for a look and finally saw there was a four-inch sign of a bicycle with a faded line through it. I had to be less than a foot away to see it. I wanted to knock this guy on his ass. I am quite certain that if I'd had a friend with me they would have done it for me! But I swallowed my anger and said, "I'm not blind, but I don't see that well." He sarcastically replied, "How convenient for you. You see just fine! What do you ride by, Braille? Yeah, you see just fine." I held it together and simply said, "I live near these trails and have for eight years. Thank you for pointing out my mistake, and I assure you that you did your good deed for the day. Now go on and finish your run and get home safely." He stared at me, confused, and I rode away, thinking about my 16 years of martial arts training and what I could do to that guy if I wanted to. Believe me, I wanted to. But I'm glad I didn't. The fear I felt just taking those first few pedal strokes was hard enough to overcome, but I felt so free and relieved that I was taking a huge step into a larger world — a world I, and others close to me, deemed unlikely if not impossible. The last thing I needed was to be challenged by an insensitive person on a trail. That first ride took every bit of courage I had.

The next ride in many ways was far, far worse, even though there were no threatening runners looking for a fight. I went up to the mountains with several friends to ride what they said was an easy trail. I figured that at least one of them would ride with me, which I thought was the plan. But few people understand that I *do* need help, even when I ask for it. To be fair, I really didn't ask for help, as I had no idea what I could or could not see. My friends took off on their bikes and I did my best, but I couldn't see anything on the trail. I crashed and crashed again. I hit trees, rocks, you name it, and fell multiple times. I lost it and shed several tears. I had finally found my limitations and I was distraught. Eventually I caught up with the group and told my friend and coaching colleague, Scott Fliegelman, that I had gone too far by adding mountain biking to my repertoire. For the rest of the day, he had me ride close behind him as he called out as many obstacles as he could. I had the time of my life. It was amazing! We made it down the trail safely, without a single crash.

Though emotionally exhausted, I had a slightly different perspective now and rethought my limitations. *Limitations.* It feels like a four-letter word to my head and heart and gives me chills to hear.

I have since worked hard to overcome my fears and have learned the proper technique to train and race off road. It's rare that I fall on my face while running on trails. It still happens, but I am better at picking myself up and going on. I have taught myself how to both run and ride primarily by *feel.* I am happy to share these techniques with anyone interested, and encourage you to contact me. There's no need for you to put yourself in danger and learn the hard way when you can benefit from the techniques that I learned. The hardest part is to not look down at what is right in front of you. It causes horrible posture and will eventually lead to injury, which I have to remind myself many times a day!

I have now raced in three Xterra races, including the World Championship in Maui. My first

Xterra was the Mountain Championship Cup in Beaver Creek, Colorado, hardly a baby step. I was fortunate to have Ivy Koger, a veteran Xterra athlete and good friend, race this with me. The bike portion of this race scared me because it plays to all of my visual weaknesses. We decided that our goal was just to finish this race as unscathed as possible. I had no business attempting to be competitive. I had a couple of crashes. Instead of giving me sympathy, Ivy treated me like any other athlete, saying, "This is mountain biking. Get up, and let's finish this!" And we did.

As for the World Championship in Maui, it was one of the most rewarding experiences of my life. I was most certainly pushed beyond my visual limitations. It was scary, technical and challenging, both physically and emotionally. It really forced me to accept that I have to adjust to my identity change. For the third time now, I have been called to the podium to share the stage with some incredible athletes. These are the athletes who fall under the heading "physically challenged," most of whom are amputees of some sort. I still have not truly realized that I am one of these fantastic people. It is just a bit confusing to me. I don't wear a prosthetic device, yet they could not be more supportive of my effort.

I have already discussed how my vision is different in different light conditions. Clearly mountain biking and trail running put me in perilous conditions, since I have blind spots in my central vision. Then there's that contrast thing again. Contrast: How do I explain *that* one to people? As you can see, it is all very confusing and I am still forced to explain my condition. But I am happy to do so, as it increases awareness of the various RDDs and how they affect people.

As I said, the other Xterra athletes at the World Championship could not have been more supportive. In fact, one of my heroes, Megan Fisher (a lower-leg amputee and the only female *in the world* with her condition who races in off-road triathlons) ended up guiding me for much of the bike course after my guide, Jared

Berg, had a major mechanical issue when his bike lost a crank arm. But being the driven athlete he is, he pushed through, using one leg to move the "working" crank and running up most of the hills carrying or pushing his bike. He got us both through the day and never gave up. He wanted me to have a great experience, and we did! Perhaps a little slower than planned, but we made it and we ran ourselves into third place in a World Championship.

I'm quite certain that Meg realized before I did what Jared was dealing with, given those bike mechanical issues, and she helped me as much as possible. But in the end, she had her own race to run. She eventually left Jared and me in the bike stage to start her run.

When we finally started our run we needed a little motivation and relief from being off the bike. The first thing I said to Jared was, "We have some runners to pick off. Let's count them off as we pass them." As we gained on our first runner (merely a shape moving in the distance), I asked Jared, "Is that a runner?" He reluctantly replied, "Yep, but it's Meg." Megan, who goes by "Peg Leg Meg," was moving right along, but alas, "Mikey Magoo" couldn't see her prosthetic device. In fact, earlier that day I had failed to recognize her and she'd told me, "You bastard, you passed me at Xterra USA Champs [the previous race] and didn't say hi." This speaks to her sense of humor. She was incredibly supportive during the bike and made it fun. She gave me words of encouragement such as "I'm proud of you, you look strong!" I would reply in my own manner with things such as "Thank you, but how does my butt look?" This made the bike portion much more pleasant and less scary. It also took my mind off Jared's bike woes. So as we came up to her, I said hi and promptly complimented her on her progress and how good she looked. I have learned that my compliments on appearance don't carry much weight, because most people discount them as "coming from a blind guy." But Meg definitely understood that I was there with some sort of vision issue, and she knew exactly what to do and what not to do. I find that very few people understand this. She made that day very special for me and I am forever grateful.

The reason I make so much of this particular experience (come on, I race a lot! This is what I do) is because in off-road races I compete in a new category. I noted the various categories above. Most people who don't race for a living compete in divisions that are grouped by age. This is how I race in most triathlons and Ironman races, but for off-road races I race in the "physically challenged/visually challenged" division. It's a new identity for me, one that I struggle with. I spend much time talking to myself, saying, "Accept it, Michael. You can't see as other athletes do, and you need help. They don't."

Should you desire to learn more about Xterra racing, visit www.xterraplanet.com. The Xterra group strongly supports challenged athletes of all kinds. I feel very fortunate that they have given me this opportunity. Although I did have to qualify for the national and world championship races by winning my division at the Beaver Creek race, Xterra has many races that *anyone* can sign up for. I hope that more visually challenged athletes will give this a try. It is well worth it and I am happy to help you on your way.

The reconstruction of my life is a work in progress. After our diagnosis with an RDD, we all go through some sort of reevaluation of life. It can be a young girl with Leber's congenital amaurosis (LCA), a teenager with Stargardt's, a college student who just realized the "walls" are closing in because of the effects of retinitis pigmentosa — the list goes on. Whatever the symptoms, change is forced upon us and we need to adjust and adapt so that we can live to our fullest.

One of the greatest lessons I have learned is also one of the most challenging: allowing others to help me. I have learned that one of the best gifts you can give another person is to allow them to help *you*. As strange as this might seem, it can do wonders for your soul as well as for those who love you most. We cannot go through this alone. Although asking for help may be terrifying, the rewards are enormous.

At some point we all deal with the shock of despair. The emotional pain associated with losing our sight is acute and needs to be faced. I tried denial, but the cruelties of nature always win. The changed life that follows will be a true test of your spirit and ability to grow. How we counteract our emotional pain will be unique. How we develop a sense of satisfaction will define our ability to endure.

I am only one of several triathletes who have visual challenges. There are not many of us, but I am hopeful that more visually impaired people will join this sport after reading this book. I am often asked what techniques I use to swim, bike and run with vision challenges. My answer? It depends on the day, the light, the road conditions, the route and several other factors. There are some constants, however. Swimming in a pool is relatively easy. Although I know it frustrates others in the pool that I cannot see the time clock, I generally use a stopwatch. I ask others in my swim lane to tell me when to go, and I hit the timer. I follow the blue or black line on the bottom and there is a nice "T" mark telling me when to make my tumble turn. No doubt I miss the wall from time to time on my turns. The toughest part of that is the embarrassment I feel when it happens. Of course, swimming in open water is a significantly greater challenge. It is more trial and error than anything else. During races I do my best to swim outside the crowd. This creates a longer swim for me, but it's far less stressful than following the buoy line that the masses tend to follow. Some courses do not allow for this, but I do my best to figure out an alternative method so that I can compete safely.

Cycling too is a significant challenge, as this is where safety takes on a greater priority. I prefer roads that have high contrast. Dark roads made from tar, with obvious and clear painted lines, are the best. Light concrete roads are extremely difficult for me to ride on, as road hazards are far less visible. I focus on a small moving target, and this continues throughout the entire ride. Cycling is further complicated by the constant need to maintain proper posture and technique. The focus this technique requires is an enormous challenge. My weekly long ride can be up to seven hours in duration. This is just one of four or five cycling sessions I do each week. Staring at pavement for seven hours, while trying to fight off negative thoughts and fear, is extremely demanding. Most people think the duration of the ride itself is exhausting — and it is — but controlling my thoughts is far more tiresome. I just can't risk taking my eyes off the road. Most cyclists look far off in the distance, see road hazards, and plan how to avoid them. But my vision doesn't allow me to see beyond just a few feet ahead of me, and I have only a split second in which to see an obstacle and avoid it or cope with not being able to avoid it.

In mountain biking, my ability to see an obstacle and avoid it is almost zero. I generally hit an obstacle and rely on technique to get me over or around it. This technique is a work in progress, but I have been very lucky so far. Of course this means I limit my speed limits to keep myself safe. I live in the mountains of Colorado, where climbing long hills is a favorite training course. Climbing hills is perfect for me, as it slows things down and helps build much-needed strength. However, as Newton's law dictates, what goes up must come down! I have to descend hills cautiously. The tires we use on road bikes are extremely thin and don't react well to even the smallest of stones, sand and the various things many motorists leave in the road. I have seen even fully sighted cyclists have deadly accidents on these roads. If *they* miss these obstacles, I think it best that I go slowly.

When racing, I am very thankful when I finish the bike stage and have started the run. Although running tends to be the greatest abuse on the human body, I love it. I use a similar technique to cycling, where I keep a strong gaze on what is right in front of me and simply react by feel. With my short-sighted gaze, however, I am still going to miss many obstacles. Skilled runners tell me that I have the least amount of head movement they have ever seen. Well, I practice a lot! I have fantastic trails just out my back door. Trail running is the most dangerous for me, given the number of rocky obstacles. Believe it or not, it is not the rocks that concern me the most — it's the rattlesnakes that blend in with the ground! While I have sprained my ankles hundreds of times and had my share of falls, I'm more concerned about getting bitten by a snake I step on because I can't see it. That's where I lose my sense of humor. Fortunately snakebites are very rare, but they do happen.

Running on roads poses different problems, which don't include rattlesnakes. Runners with vision concerns similar to mine tell me that potholes are their greatest challenge. I agree!

What's Next?

Although hundreds of thousands of dollars were raised for FFB through my racing events, I felt that I needed to do more to increase awareness and raise funds for blindness research, as well as to help others learn life skills to cope with their low vision. "What's next?" I wondered. Eventually, this led me to two new projects: creating the Race to Cure Blindness and writing *Eye Envy*.

I asked all the people featured in this book what inspires them. For every interview I do, I ask that same darn question! But when someone asks it of *me,* it consistently causes me to hesitate, as I never really have a complete answer.

I guess part of the answer is that I'm self-motivated. But that still doesn't answer the question. When I think back to my childhood, I always feel that it's full of unfinished business. I think of all those physical education classes where I took every opportunity to avoid participating, and if I did participate, I was nearly the last person picked for a team, which never felt good. Somewhere along the line I tapped into my inner athlete that I hadn't known existed. I think about this often during those ridiculously long training sessions as well as on race days. Racing is a metaphor for life, condensed into one day. Throughout the long miles of swimming, cycling and running, there are many ups and downs. For every down, an up is around the corner, and of course the opposite also holds true. It's how we deal with the down moments that carries us to that finish line and gains us satisfaction.

Thank you for allowing me to share my story with you.

chapter 2

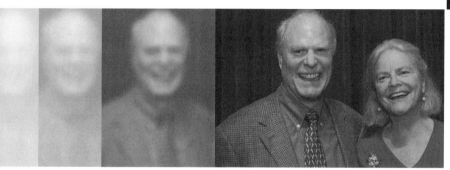

gordon gund

Co-founder and chairman of the
Foundation Fighting Blindness;
philanthropist; entrepreneur; family man;
diagnosed with retinitis pigmentosa

Introduction

I feel honored that Gordon agreed to participate in *Eye Envy*. By helping found and fund
the Foundation Fighting Blindness, Gordon
has contributed greatly to finding treatments
and cures for those with "all" retinal degenerative diseases. Although he is blind, he has
accomplished more than anyone else I know.

I first met Gordon at a private dinner at FFB's
Day of Science in January 2006. The dinner guests included my parents and me, Bill
Schmidt (the Foundation's chief executive of-
ficer), Gordon and his wife, Lulie, and the Mc-
Nallys. I was told the McNallys are the McNal-
ly half of the famed map-making corporation
Rand-McNally. Although I was the subject of
the Foundation Fighting Blindness's 2006 an-
nual-report cover story, I was anxious about
meeting this high-powered businessman and
co-founder of FFB. I was also nervous about
being with someone who is so visually challenged, as I still did not understand these diseases and how those affected by them coped

with their effects.

My parents and I were both honored and confused by our invitation to socialize with these heavy hitters: We wondered, "Why have we warranted this dinner invitation?" I couldn't keep my eyes off Gordon. I watched as he dined while conversing with the other guests on a wide range of topics in a way that was interesting and informed, but not arrogant. Gordon asked me if I skied, since I live in Colorado. I told him that I had made the difficult decision to stop skiing, as it was such a struggle with the glare hindering me from enjoying a sport I loved so much. However, he encouraged me to continue skiing with the help of guides, as he did.

Gordon selflessly devotes hours of his time raising funds for the Foundation Fighting Blindness. We are blessed to have his energy and influence working for us. When I read Gordon's story, I feel like I'm receiving a lesson about how scientists are working to solve vision loss, as well as learning about the devastating emotional and physical effects of vision loss. We all owe him gratitude for sharing his story with us. Our gratitude is best expressed by doing everything we can to help him in his efforts.

Gordon Gund's Story

The year 1965 was very important for me for several reasons. It was when I met my future wife, Lulie Liggett, whom I married in 1966. But it was also when I began to experience relative difficulty seeing at night. I say "relative" because I may have been losing peripheral vision many years before that, due to an inherited eye disease called retinitis pigmentosa. Typically, RP causes peripheral vision loss that's most noticeable at first at night, but gradually also is noticeable during the day. However, at the time I didn't know that I had RP and that my vision probably was never what would be considered "good." The fact that I was noticing changes, though, made me start trying to find out what was going on.

For many months I did not have an accurate diagnosis. It was only in 1966 when I had a test called an electroretinagram, or ERG, that I was told that I had this thing called retinitis pigmentosa, which would cause me to lose more and more of my sight both at night and eventually during the day. The doctor said that it was likely I would keep useful vision until my 60s. I was then 26, and 60 seemed awfully far away. The doctors told me there was nothing I could do to stop or change the disease, so I went ahead with working at Chase Manhattan Bank and attending New York University and of course, enjoying Lulie's and my wonderful new marriage. However, I did try to limit the impact my decreasing night vision was having on my ability to do things.

In November of 1966, my father died rather suddenly at the age of 79. He had been the best man at my wedding and was a dominant figure in my life. I revered him, and had just really gotten to know him as a friend. This was a huge loss to me, but I will discuss more about "loss" later.

In March 1968, Lulie and I celebrated the birth of our first child, Grant. Just a little later I left Chase Manhattan Bank to start a new venture capital company in New York. We moved to Princeton and I commuted in and out of New York by train. As my night vision grew steadily worse, getting to and from the trains in Princeton and New York after dark became quite difficult. In 1969 I had to give up driving at night, which was a big loss of independence. I was only 29. I was very concerned about what else was in store. I also was having increasing difficulty seeing at night while on foot, and even during the day I noticed big changes when I walked from sunlight into dimly lit buildings.

By early 1970, my night vision was all but gone. I also began to notice a real deterioration of my day vision. I went from being able to read paragraphs at a time, to sentences, then to words and then only single letters. All of that happened within about six months. Of course, I had to give up flying, which I had still been able to do during daylight hours, and more importantly, I had to be careful even when walking. When my day vision started to go I became very worried, even frantic. With Lulie's help, I searched for some form of treatment or a way to stop the progression of the disease. Time after time we encountered dead ends. Throughout that summer, I was depressed and frustrated, as bit by bit my field of vision was blurring out to darkness and there seemed to be no treatments available. Our second child, Zachary, was born in October 1970 and that gave me a tremendous emotional lift, although by then I only had narrow tunnel vision and was barely able to see him.

Earlier that year, I had heard that the Russians had a treatment for retinitis pigmentosa. Although American scientists and medical doctors didn't hold out much hope for its success, as the treatment had no basis in science, I nevertheless decided to try it.

Five weeks after Zack's birth, and just two weeks after the last of my remaining vision was gone, I received a visa to go to Soviet

Russia. Since Lulie was nursing our new-born and couldn't travel, my brother Graham agreed to accompany me to the Filotov Institute in Odessa, where I was expecting a four-day treatment. The Filotov Institute was a Russian Revolution-era eye hospital that was in terrible disrepair. I was assigned a bed in a small room that housed six other patients who were much older than I, and spoke no English. In fact, other than the woman who headed the institute, no one else at the institute understood or spoke English. Making matters worse, I was told the treatment would take four *weeks*, not four days! Graham could only stay for a week before he had to return to his new architectural business in Boston, and even during the time he was in Odessa he rarely was allowed to visit me. Since I spoke no Russian, and by then couldn't see to use sign language, I was essentially isolated. Capping off my isolation, there was no telephone service for calling the United States.

Though Lulie and I were unable to communicate for many weeks, I realized that feeling sorry for myself was not going to do me any good. And, although the Russian treatment did nothing to improve my vision, being isolated for those long weeks forced me to accept that I was now blind, which I had been denying and fighting for a long time. At the institute I didn't need to pretend that I could see, nor deny that I was blind. As the treatments progressed without any success, I had to accept the fact of my condition.

In Russia, I decided to focus on what I *could* do, not focus on what I could not. I realized that I didn't want blindness to change how I lived my life or affect my relationships with Lulie, Grant or Zack. I wanted our lives to be as full as possible, which could be achieved only if I didn't allow my disability to limit me.

Most people know what it is to suffer a loss such as the death of a relative or friend, or even a pet. When that happens, you're overcome with sadness and grief, but over time the grief and mourning lessen and you are able to go for days or weeks without being reminded of the loved one who died. But when you suffer the loss of a physical sense or capability, such as your sight, the mourning never really resolves. It's a living loss, one that you confront daily as you try to re-invent your world without being able to see. You never forget how that sense or faculty used to help orient you in the world.

For those of us who have a disease that erases our sight, not dwelling on the negative takes not just *our* determination, it also takes the determination and caring of the people around us — in my case, Lulie, Grant and Zack. Our family and friends have to believe in us, support us and deal with us when we are frustrated and down. I know that in the years since I've lost my eyesight, there have been many frustrating times. As much as I struggle against it, I grieve that I'm not able to see and do what I used to. I miss being able to see the people I love, my family and friends. I miss the beautiful sunsets and sunrises, and every ordinary thing that people with normal sight can see whenever they like. When that happens I get down and frustrated. There are things I naturally would like to be able to do; I'm sure that's true for everyone. Sometimes just doing the things I want to do takes a lot more time, energy and thought than it would if I could see.

Now let me go back to 1970 just once more, because in addition to the great highlight of Zack's birth and, in a way, my own rebirth, I also had a chance to meet Jim Wheat, who is a role model for me. Months before Zack's birth and my trip to Russia, Lulie and I traveled to Richmond, Virginia, to see a doctor who reportedly had been working a treatment for RP. When I asked him about his research and whether or not he'd found anything that could stop the progress of RP, he told me that unfortunately he had reached a dead end with his research. This was devastating to me, as he was one of my last hopes. I kind of broke down at that point, saying I didn't know what I would be able to do when I went blind.

The doctor told me he knew of a local man,

Jim Wheat, who had RP and was not only the head of a regional investment banking firm and a major business force in Richmond, but also served as the financial advisor to Virginia's governor. Jim went blind at the age of 21 from RP, but still rode horseback in what is called the Deep Run Hunt. He also was very active in, and involved with, community and nonprofit events and activities. Of course I wanted to meet him right away. When the doctor called Jim, he invited Lulie and me to come right over. For much of that afternoon we sat in Jim's office high above the Rappahannock River in Richmond, while he took calls from the governor, made several trades, spoke to his son and to his wife, joined a number of investment syndicates and just conducted his usual business. He barely spoke with us the whole time, but allowed us to witness a typical day in his life. Lulie and I realized that despite being blind, Jim was engaged fully in his life, which included helping others, being productive, making thoughtful decisions and, most importantly, making a real contribution to his community. When I left his office, I felt as if I was floating on air. Blindness didn't have to be "the end."

The memory of our afternoon in Jim's office has stuck with me, not only because it encouraged me to continue pursuing my own aspirations despite blindness, but because Jim allowed me and Lulie into his life in such a personal way. It has inspired me to allow others who are grieving about the loss of their sight similar access to my life when it seems appropriate. I returned temporarily to fighting the blindness that was coming on me and to trying to deny it. Long after blindness won that battle, that afternoon has stuck with me. Not only because of what it meant to me personally in terms of my own aspirations, but also what his time, the time he allowed me to be part of, meant to me. Also, what maybe I can do, from time to time and when it seems to make sense, for other people who are faced with the same kind of loss.

Also during that frenetic 1970 search for

some way to stop my impending blindness, Lulie and I met with Dr. Eliot Berson, an ophthalmologist affiliated with Harvard Medical School's Massachusetts Eye and Ear Infirmary. Dr. Berson conducted research on retinal degeneration and macular degeneration, as well as RP and Usher's syndrome, all of which are members of a family of inherited degenerative diseases of the retina. Dr. Berson was very caring in his diagnosis of me and frank about what my prognosis was. He told me he wanted to develop a multi-disciplined research laboratory for the study of retinal degeneration — he believed that there are ways to prevent, treat and even cure heritable diseases of the retina. However, at that time he had no hopeful answers for me. Lulie and I told him that someday, when we had coped with my immediate problems, we would help support his research efforts so that other retinal degenerative disease sufferers might not endure the same frustrations and dead ends that we had.

In mid-1971, we called Dr. Berson with the

news that we wanted to help him create a research facility that covered many scientific and clinical disciplines, as he had described a year earlier. Berson introduced us to the Bermans, a family with two daughters who were just beginning to lose their sight from RP, and a few other families with similar stories. By the end of that year, this group of like-minded people banded together to start the RP Foundation, which for Lulie and me was a way to take the experience we had with RP and turn it into something positive.

Over the years, the Foundation's name has changed from RP Foundation to the Foundation Fighting Blindness. The name change reflects the Foundation's research mission to understand the causes of the family of retinal degenerative diseases (RDDs), not just retinitis pigmentosa, and to treat, cure and eventually prevent RDDs so that future generations will no longer be affected by them.

From its inception, Lulie and I were co-founders and trustees of the Foundation. I was the vice-chairman and Lulie started the first chapter of the Foundation, in New Jersey. By 1974, we had raised funds for the Berman-Gund Laboratory, which studies retinal degenerations. Over the past 36 years, this Harvard Medical School-affiliated laboratory has increased our understanding of how retinal degenerative diseases affect the cells of the retina, how the visual function works, how the retina works, and even which genes are involved in some retinal degenerations. The Laboratory is now working hard on various cures and ways of slowing the progress of RDDs. Among the Laboratory's major impacts and breakthroughs was the development of a vitamin therapy that dramatically slows the progress of retinitis pigmentosa.

Since the opening of the Berman-Gund Laboratory, we at FFB have funded other research facilities in the United States and around the world. The Foundation has grown from its initial small group of founders to include thousands of people around the United States. We have 45 affiliate organizations in the U.S., and

33 other countries around the world have affiliate societies that are studying how to cure and treat RDDs. The Foundation's scientists feel positive that within the next 10 years — and perhaps within five years — we will have solutions for the more than 10 million people in the U.S., and the many millions more worldwide, who suffer from retinal degenerative diseases.

Lulie and I have been actively involved with the Foundation since it began. In 1986, I became the Foundation's chairman, in which capacity I still serve today. Lulie and I spend a lot of time with individuals and families of children who are diagnosed with RDDs. That's very important to us. As Jim Wheat did for us, we are giving back to our community, helping others and providing hope for the future.

Before I lost my sight at age 30, I was fortunate to have many good experiences that taught me teamwork, leadership, and entrepreneurial skills. I attended first-rate schools and universities, playing on high school and college-level sports teams, where I learned how important teamwork is to winning. I then served for three-and-a-half years in the Navy as an officer on a destroyer in the Western Pacific, where I learned leadership skills. My early business experience was at the Chase Manhattan Bank in New York, where I went through an intense development training pro-gram and became a commercial lending of-ficer, while also attending New York Univer-sity's Leonard N. Stern School of Business at night. While traveling for Chase, I realized that entrepreneurs were the people I wanted to work with and emulate. In 1968, I established Gund Investment Corporation, a diversified in-vestment company, and Gunwyn Ventures, a venture capital company, and worked exten-sively with the entrepreneurs whose ventures we financed.

In 1972, we at FBB convinced nine world-class scientists to volunteer their time and serve as FFB's Scientific Advisory Board to provide the expertise we sorely lacked. I went to New York and talked to the president of the National Health Agencies Council to learn more about how we should go about our mission. I was told that every year well-intended groups form foundations to fund research about various diseases, but that 98 percent of them fail. This information increased our determination to succeed. With help from many volunteers – plus some serendipity – by early 1973 the FFB had raised enough capital to fund the Berman-Gund Laboratory, which opened in 1974.

Many hundreds of volunteers helped us fundraise. We had support not only from people all around the country, but from all around the world. We determined to raise more and more money to fund more research, and we were successful. Coincidentally, the National Institutes of Health formed the National Eye Institute at about the time the Foundation was raising money for innovative research. Although the NEI only provided grants to proven, published scientists, they soon realized that the Foundation was a great training ground for researchers. Essentially, the Foundation functioned as an early-stage venture capital company for the NIH, funding innovative research. As our researchers made progress, the NEI would then take over funding their research, and the FFB would move on to funding other novel approaches, developing more innovators and researchers in the field of retinal degenerative disease.

Throughout the 1970s and into the early 1980s, most of our fundraising was done by volunteers. By 1980, we had 45 volunteer chapters around the country and affiliate societies in 33 other countries, but we had only a few administrative staff at the headquarters. By the early 80s, we had raised more than $30 million for research, had 11 research centers and another 30 or so grantees, but it was clear we were suffering from volunteer fatigue and burnout. For the years 1983 through 1985 our revenue stayed flat, which meant we weren't able to increase our funding for research. At the same time, new technologies had been developed that made it possible to identify the defective genes in hereditary diseases, so the demand for additional research funding was increasing just when we'd lost our impetus.

We realized it was time to change from a mom-and-pop-style, mostly volunteer model to a professional organization with paid staff who take their direction from the board. However, others of us didn't like the proposed changes. After some tumultuous and destructive debate, as well as some constructive imagining, some members left, and new people who are highly committed to the mission and not burdened by the Foundation's history were recruited for the board. Happily, from 1986 through 2002, we grew our revenues at a compound annual rate of growth of 12.5 percent, and the amount we put into research grew at a slightly higher rate.

The Foundation is very fortunate to have an extraordinary professional staff, but this progress could simply not have happened without two other very important groups of people: volunteers and donors at the local level, and exceptional volunteer leadership at the national level. Our volunteer base has grown to include many thousands of people. We have now raised more than $350 million for research, and the National Eye Institute has provided almost five times that amount to fund projects for which FBB provided the initial funding. In recent years, there has been an explosion in the numbers of research breakthroughs, and potentially viable therapies are emerging from the laboratory at the rate of more than one every month.

Getting research into clinics and then to patients is now our major challenge and opportunity – and it means we are once again need to change our organizational model! This time, however, an already rejuvenated board, a strong professional staff, and the Scientific Advisory Board are in agreement about what changes need to be implemented for the next round of growth. Constructive imagining is under way, and we are in the process of meeting our challenges and opportunities. It is a very exciting time for the Foundation Fighting Blindness and for the research it has been spearheading. We know it's only a matter of years before treatments and cures will be available to people here and around the world.

So, what has blindness done for me?

I've learned to be much better organized than I was when I had sight. My memory is more developed. I retain information and retrieve it better and faster than I did before blindness. I also listen to people and the world around me with intent. Now I really can hear what people are saying to me because I'm not concerned with how they look or what their mannerisms are. I really focus on and pay attention to the substance of their conversation.

My ability to be productive and effective is greatly improved, although I do take more time and energy doing the simple things — shaving, getting dressed, moving around, reading and getting information — that are fairly easy for someone who is sighted. I do have to depend on other people to help with transportation, to tell me what's going on around me so that I have situational context, and to help me with finding information that I need. I've learned to judge who will understand my limitations and who may not, and I've learned to ask people for help. That's not easy, because I want to be as independent as possible. But I've found that most people have a basic need to help others. Hopefully, my appreciation of their help is important to them, too.

To do the things I do, I must be able to get accurate information quickly. I am fortunate to have the resources to afford a reader and executive assistants in my office. I also have a driver, and in more recent years, an airplane and crew that take me more easily to far-away places. Without the wonderful people I have working with me, I would not be able to access information so fast or get around as easily as I do. I know I would still want to do as much as I could, but I don't think I would be able to do nearly as much as I do now.

Reading for me is *listening*, whether for business, for the Foundation Fighting Blindness, or other interests. If you're blind, you can't just get information when and how you want it — you have to think about what you want to learn about, and plan to get it. Listening is not as convenient or easy as reading with your eyes. Much more effort is involved. When you're listening, you can't just pause and review previous information like you can when you're reading. You have to know how to categorize what's important, while still listening to what else is being said. Listening, rather than reading, entails greater work to cover material, understand it and remember it.

This is an exciting time for the Foundation. We are growing, both in size of the organization and the amount of money we can invest annually in research. More importantly, the "rate of return" on our research investment is accelerating rapidly! We have several human clinical trials under way now, and many more that will be beginning soon. Human clinical trials test how drugs or therapies work in human subjects, and are key to getting a drug or therapy approved by the Food and Drug Administration. Without FDA approval, remedies cannot be made available to the public, so successful clinical trials are crucial to developing any drug or therapy. Many new, promising therapies are emerging from the laboratory and entering the pre-clinical pipeline at a rate of four a month, and that number is increasing.

Recent successes include the Genentech drug Lucentis, created to treat wet (or advanced) age-related macular degeneration — the research that it's based on came from work that was funded by FFB. More recently, research at the Berman-Gund Laboratory is showing that some forms of RP degeneration can be dramatically slowed by using certain nutritional supplements.

Why is all this research so important? Retinal degenerative diseases affect more than 10 million Americans and many times that number worldwide. The leading cause of blindness for Americans over 55 years old is age-related macular degeneration. It's estimated to affect over 1.6 million Americans, and this number will increase greatly as the baby boomer generation reaches 55 and older. Other inheritable retinal degenerative diseases include retinitis pigmentosa, which affects over 200,000 people in the U.S., and Usher's syndrome, which causes both blindness and deafness. These diseases are hereditary or have an inherited component, they are all progressive or degenerative, and they are all retinal – that is, they cause the light-receiving retinal cells, known as photoreceptors or rods and cones, to die. The retina is the part of the eye that is attached directly to the central nervous system. It is actually separated from the rest of the eye by the blood-brain barrier. The retina is the only part of the brain that can be seen from outside the body, by looking through the pupil into the back of the eye's structure. Research done to cure retinal diseases may also help scientists understand how to treat and prevent other neurodegenerative diseases that involve the central nervous system, such as Alzheimer's disease and multiple sclerosis. This may well be an additional significant benefit to the already very important work to fight blindness.

Author's note: Chapter 15 has updated information about research and treatments for all the diseases covered in Eye Envy. *In the time since I interviewed Gordon, there have been even more breakthroughs!*

Most importantly, to conclude Gordon's story, I want to emphasize something I wrote in my introduction: Gordon and Lulie have very little reason to make both the financial and time investment for this cause. This as close to true altruism as I have ever seen. I know that Gordon is proud of his efforts, but won't be completely satisfied until these cures and treatments for RDDs are part of everyday practice. He is an inspiration to me personally and to millions more.

chapter 3

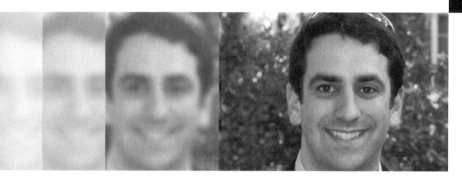

jeremy block

Ph.D. in biochemistry; M.A. in public policy; athlete; spokesperson for the visually impaired; teacher; mentor; diagnosed with cone-rod dystrophy and one hell of a sense of humor!

Introduction

Talking one day with Charlie Kelly, one of my Boulder friends, I told him I was writing a book that guides people after they've been diagnosed with a retinal degenerative disease. "I have a friend from college who has a disease called cone-rod dystrophy," said Charlie. "Wow!" I said. "That's the same disease I have — it's quite rare." I'd met only a few other people who had it, and I wanted to meet Charlie's friend. And that's how I came to know Jeremy Block, although as I write this book, Jeremy and I have never met face to face.

After one brief conversation with Jeremy, I knew he would be an essential part of this project. He has more to offer the entire low-vision community than almost anyone else. His accomplishments speak for themselves, but his passion for changing the world is amazing and encouraging. He is incredibly energetic. His story is particularly interesting because he knew of his disease from birth. Although he didn't have to deal with a long diagnosis process as others typically do, he still had to cope with all the same challenges of being visually challenged in a sighted world. The difference here is that he has actually done something about it that will benefit us all.

I take great pride in having Jeremy's participation in this book, as I share many of his conclusions about public policy as it relates to those who are disabled and how to make the most of our disability. I especially love how Jeremy has taken the close influences of those around him and allowed these relationships to help shape his life, both educationally and professionally. I found it both illuminating and emotional to hear Jeremy's story – I wish I had met him years ago. He could have made my adaptive process far more pleasant. In fact, I hope that all the stories in this book encourage you and show you ways of coping and adapting to life with vision challenges, to make your process easier.

You would be hard-pressed to find someone more passionate about this cause than Jeremy. He and I frequently discuss fairly heavy topics. His perspective is powerful and has helped me see many aspects of life in a different manner. He has helped me rise above my own perspective. Much of Jeremy's story goes way beyond just telling the facts about his life. He gives us insights that he has learned and cultivated in a very profound way. Please enjoy Jeremy's story.

Jeremy Block's Story

I was born with cone-rod dystrophy. Well, at least that is what I've been told. At one point I think a piece of paper from an ophthalmologist I trust said it was "just" cone dystrophy, but now I am pretty sure he was half correct and it affects my rods as well. It isn't his fault, he is very good at his job, but I see out of these eyes and he doesn't. I have a degenerative eye disorder that has a genetic component to it. The genetic component is that my mother has the same problem, and her father did as well. The name and nature of the disorder only matter in one fundamental way: how I respond to it and adapt to the rather unique challenges it presents me with.

My Role Models

My parents and my sister are exceptional people. Their unconditional love, guidance and support are key ingredients to my success. Their backgrounds and what they've achieved inspire me. My grandparents also play a significant role in my life.

My "legally blind" mother was a social worker for the Department of Social Services in the county where I grew up. She retired on disability because she has the same eye condition as I do. She then went back after retiring from public service to get a doctoral degree studying grandparent-grandchild relationships. She has always been civic minded, and served on interfaith coalitions and helped provide food to those in need by starting a food pantry. She is one of the most enthusiastic and high-energy people I know.

My father is a retired police officer. He was a sergeant in the sheriff's department in the county where I grew up. He sacrificed mightily for my family, working the night shift in a very difficult environment. He worked overtime so that he and my mother could live in a decent neighborhood and my sister and I would have some money saved for college. He is humble and soft-spoken, but incredibly bright and insightful. Both of my parents stressed the importance of school and encouraged my sister and me to get jobs while growing up so we could know what it meant to put in a day's work. They instilled in us a strong sense of faith, a firm commitment to public service, and showered us with the perfect kind of love. Their love wasn't overly coddling or sheltering. If we did well and had success we celebrated; if we did poorly, they explained why we didn't succeed and encouraged us to get better while trying to provide us the means to improve. Lastly, they grew with us becoming our closest friends. This last part is what I cherish the most.

My grandmother Betty passed away when I was very young. My love for her has grown through stories and the impact she had on her husband, Henry, and their children.

My grandfather Henry was born in 1923 on the kitchen table in their section of Brooklyn, New York. The son of Eastern European immigrants, he grew up during the Great Depression, excelled in school and attended the prestigious Brooklyn Technical High School. He then enlisted in the Army and was a master sergeant in World War II, and was among the first groups to enter the city of Hiroshima, Japan, after the atomic bomb was dropped on that city. After the war, he returned and started a family. He worked for the Department of the Navy at the Brooklyn Navy Yard and moved to a few other places while my father and uncle were growing up. By the time I was born in 1980, my grandfather was living on Long Island, New York. When I was a sophomore in high school we convinced him to move up to near where we lived in Syracuse. This was great for me, because my grandfather shares my curiosity for electronics and mechanical devices. Also, he and I have a great way of communicating with one another by making faces and nudging or poking one another. We can sit for hours on end laughing and discussing without actually speaking.

My grandparents Rose and Aaron lived near me throughout my childhood. Aaron had the same vision problem that my mother and I have. Unfortunately, he passed away from lung cancer when I was only in the sixth grade. At that age I was not old enough to ask him how he coped with this eye disorder as he grew up. However, my geographically inconsistent love for the Dallas Cowboys came from my grandfather Aaron. I still don't know why he was a Cowboys fan, but I am one because of him. In general, I've mostly come to know him through my grandmother Rose and my mom.

I was in elementary school when the Americans with Disabilities Act passed and we, as a nation, formally said we had to stop discrimination against people with disabilities. It turned my school experience into one where I was not only the first child to be testing the waters in certain situations with how the practical implementation of this law would go for my own education, but it would set up precedents for the students who followed. I guess this might be one of the places where I developed my active desire to be a trailblazer. I started attending my own Individual Education Plan (IEP) meetings in middle school within a year of when the ADA passed. This was circa 1992-'93. Some teachers thought it was a wonderful idea for me to attend them; others were appalled that they had to say what they thought of me to my face

Growing up with this disorder did many things to me. I learned some things much earlier and in a much harsher way than my classmates did. I didn't realize it then, but most students don't have to learn that some teachers think disabled children cannot succeed as adults. That's a very harsh lesson to learn at a young age. On the other hand, I've had several teachers readily admit that having me in their class made them better teachers because it forced them to think more creatively and broadly about what it really meant to teach. In a few instances I was lucky enough to see how I changed the lives of others, and that went a long way towards making the tough lessons, such as learning that a teacher doesn't believe you'll succeed, a little easier to deal with.

I was only sometimes treated well by my classmates, but most treated me poorly. For much of my schooling, I was upset and didn't respond well to being treated so poorly. It was a messy time for me. I was struggling to understand what I could and couldn't see or do, all the while trying to develop the appropriate skills for coping with schoolmates who would torment anyone who was different from them.

The Teacher-Student Relationship

Teachers play an important role in young people's lives. The most important things I learned from my teachers are: long-term consistency, tough love, figuring out when other people count as teachers, and realizing that I am a teacher, too.

Long-term consistency: Having a few teachers who you develop a close and lasting relation-ship with is critically important and life enrich-ing. I've had two long-term teachers in my life. The first is Donna Richards, my teacher for the visually impaired (TVI), and the second is James Morgan, my high school chemistry teacher.

It was during elementary school that Donna Richards identified me. She went by the nick-name RJ then (at the time her last name was Richards-Johnson. From the first day I met her until today, she's been a constant in my life. She taught me how to advocate for myself and supported every decision I made in my educa-tion. More importantly, she encouraged me to reciprocate by helping younger disabled students who followed in my footsteps.

Since high school, I have met with younger students in my school district who have visual impairments. Growing up, I always wished that I had someone older than myself who had gone through it all and could answer my questions. So, despite no longer living in the area, I try to return once a year to meet with Donna's students. I count this as one of the most fulfilling things I get to do.

When I return to the Syracuse area, I have a full day of visiting with these students. Donna and I start in the morning and go from school to school. I get a good 20-to-30-minute session with each student. Afterwards, we usually discuss how the day went. After doing this over a period of years, I see students grow up; I have snapshots of where their lives have taken them. I take pride in the fact that many of them are navigating the system with far fewer stumbling blocks than I encountered.

In high school I met James Morgan, a fantastic chemistry teacher. He was in his first year teaching at my school when I took honors chemistry. He knows exactly how to connect with students and get them excited about chemistry. He accommodated my vision disability by having me help set up all the labs for class a day before each lab was taught.

During setup, I'd do the lab myself with Mr. Morgan instructing me. The next day when we did the lab in class, I didn't have to worry about problems with seeing things and wouldn't require extra assistance. In fact, doing each lab twice helped me learn the material so well that I got all A's in the course. And it counted as my service hours for the New York State Science Honor Society, so it worked out really well. That's a dedicated teacher!

The most fun I had in high school chemistry was a demonstration we did to show reactivity of certain elements. We had a large beaker full of water underneath the protective hood. We then had small amounts of pure sodium and potassium. He allowed me to drop pieces of each into the water. The subsequent explosion sounded like a shotgun, and my lab partner, Liz, let out the loudest shriek I've ever heard. The neighboring teachers ran down the hall and thought something had gone wrong. It was hilarious! I knew then that I wanted to be a scientist. Granted, I think my parents knew I was destined to be a scientist a long time before that.

I also return to my old high school and talk with Mr. Morgan and his classes. I answer questions for them about what kinds of careers people can pursue in the sciences and what options are available to students if they major in chemistry or biology in college, and what sorts of programs are available for graduate study in the physical and life sciences in the United States. Mr. Morgan still does many of the same demonstrations, and his students like him and his teaching style just as much as I did.

Tough love: In the safe environment of the school, tough love from some of my teachers prepared me for the harsh realities of how others might, and in some cases did, treat me.

In elementary school my second grade teacher Mrs. Finkelstein scolded me once for raising my voice to another student who would taunt me by calling me "blind as a bat." I will never forget how hard on me she was about it. She made it clear that I was never to let others get the best of me with their mean words.

In middle school, I was frustrated because several days a week during what should be my recess time, I had to meet with Donna and learn how to touch-type. My sixth-grade social studies and math teacher, Mr. O, was known to be a tough teacher. I remember complaining to him that it wasn't fair that the other kids got to play outside every day, while many days during recess I had to sit inside and do more lessons. He was pretty unapologetic about it and told me that some people will just have to work harder for the same things. By the end of the year I could touch-type, and I was typing reports for his class on a computer, something that few other students did at that time.

Toward the end of middle school, I had one teacher in particular who taught me a very harsh lesson. I will be charitable and say he was using tough love. Mr. Stokes was a social studies teacher widely known as a student favorite, but I could sense he didn't like me. In my IEP meeting that year, Mr. Stokes told my parents and the other teachers that he thought I was faking my vision problem. Needless to say, I didn't feel like working hard in his class after that. Just because someone is beloved by many others doesn't mean they are always right or always treat people well. Not everyone that people look up to is squeaky clean.

Author's note: This is an experience that many of us with vision disabilities face. It was a common theme for many of the hundreds of people I interviewed.

In high school I had two teachers in particular that dished out a fair bit of tough love. The first was Mr. McGuigan, my social studies teacher, who kicked me out of class many times for talking back to him. The only problem is, I was getting straight A's in his class! It was too easy for me and at the end of the year I got one of the highest grades on the final exam of anyone. I deserved the discipline and I imagine that I was a real pain to deal with.

Similarly, in my sophomore biology course Mr. Searle counseled me daily and helped me troubleshoot the labs for the class that required drawing out what we observed and identifying important components. This was difficult for me, and he really did a marvelous job of making the class and the material accessible.

However, every once in a while I would act up in class. He finally told me in his booming voice to leave the room and not come back, because I kept interrupting him. At the time, I had been asking him to read something from the blackboard because I couldn't see it — normally he read things aloud for me. Later, after class, he sat me down to explain why he had punished me, and told me about the importance of keeping order in the classroom. He said that he wanted to show me that people could be unreasonable. He expected someday I would be treated that way, and he wanted me to learn how to respond to it in a safe environment so that I would know how to cope with unreasonable people in other situations.

Teachers can come in many forms, and from the most unexpected places. But we have to be able to recognize when an unconventional teacher pops into our lives, and be willing to learn from him or her. In college, the captain of my cross-country team was a guy named Charlie (Chuck) Kelly. Chuck is an all-American kind of guy. He grew up in Iowa, attended Duke on a Navy ROTC scholarship, and ran track and cross-country. He kept his nose clean and worked incredibly hard. We referred to Chuck as "the horse," and I count him as one of the best people I met in college. What I admired about Chuck in college was how he balanced his commitments, while still making meaningful connections with people. He was one of the few people who really took the time to understand what I faced with my eye problems.

What I didn't know for a while is that Chuck has a sibling who has a cognitive disability. I think that the love he has for his family and knowing how hard it can be to navigate this world when you have an extra layer of barriers due to a disability is one of those shared understandings that strengthened our friendship. The good news is that there are a lot of people in this world with that understanding, and it's a piece of common ground that we all can build on. That's what Chuck taught me, and for that I'm forever grateful.

Another pair of teachers, in both a formal and informal sense, are David and Jane Richardson. They are my Ph.D. advisors. They jointly run the laboratory and are two peas in a pod. They have integrated their lives and work together, which is inspiring.

I first met the Richardsons when I was an undergraduate. I took a course from them. After I described to them my visual limitations, they worked closely with me to ensure that I could succeed in their class. I was so intrigued by the research they do that I asked them if I could work in their lab one summer. That began a long-standing friendship and working relationship. The two of them discern the world differently from most people, and I think that my visual impairment has made me evaluate the world differently as well. They've taught me that it's not a problem to literally or figuratively see the world differently from other people. With the Richardsons' help, I've turned my sight differences into a strength: I now believe that what I actually see are the truly important elements. I'm much more able to pick out the important information that I see and identify it. For my research, which ironically includes 3-D visualization, I'm able to design representations of the most important information for understanding my area of scientific research. The bottom line is that if I can see it and understand it, then chances are just about anyone else can too!

When I started to become interested not just in the details of my scientific research, but also the societal implications of science, I began working on the Institutional Review Board (IRB) at Duke Medicine. The goal of the IRB is to oversee research that has humans as subjects, and ensure that their rights are being protected. It was a great opportunity for me to blend together my interest in the rights of people with disabilities with the science that I had been learning at Duke both as an undergraduate and a graduate student. This work really helped put the bug in me for participating in public service. Towards that end, I applied and was accepted into Duke's Master of Public Policy degree program (MPP) to go along with my Ph.D. degree in biochemistry.

In the MPP program I met a great professor named Tom Taylor. Tom is a North Carolina native who spent most of his career working in the Department of Defense in Washington, D.C. He's one of the most polished and gifted lecturers I came across at Duke. I took courses from him on national security, public management, and leadership. He's a consummate gentleman and is genuinely interested in the development of young people who are interested in public service. Through many discussions over a few years, one of the things that Tom has helped me to learn is how to integrate different perspectives into a narrative that people can understand. This is incredibly important, not only for what I want to do in my career, but also for the everyday issues I face as a person with a visual impairment. Being able to take a lot of information and present it in just the right way to get your point across is both an art and a science. Tom taught me how to explain to the general public, in 30 seconds or less, what are the barriers visually impaired people face and how they can partner with other visually impaired people to overcome those barriers. That's an incredibly useful accomplishment!

Before I started the MPP program, I met a professor named Bob Cook-Deegan. One of the best things I've learned from Bob is that it is OK to have a nonlinear career path. Bob got a chemistry degree from Harvard University, a medical degree from the University of Colorado, was a molecular biology researcher, and then held various policy-related positions both in and out of government. He's written one of the definitive histories of the Human Genome Project, appropriately titled *The Gene Wars*. When I was considering getting my MPP I met with Bob. Like my Ph.D. advisors, he recognized that I could go in a nontraditional direction with my degree, and has supported me since day one. He's helped guide me in my pursuits and has given me honest feedback on what I'm doing so that I can always improve. I value his mentoring and think that having a strong relationship with my mentors is critical to my success. They can teach you not only how to navigate your career, but they can teach you what traps to avoid and encourage you to keep striving to do better. Mentors serve as your own personal cheerleaders as well as your most effective teachers.

In the summer of 2008, I interned at a federal agency, the Office of Management and

Budget (OMB). The unit where I interned had a cast of characters who turned out to be incredible teachers! Gene Ebner, my boss and chief of the branch, along with Dick Feezle, a co-worker with a lot of experience, taught me more in three months about public service and how the government works than I think most people have the opportunity to learn over their entire career. Gene and Dick invited me into a whole new world. They let me do substantive work, gave me advice, and made me a part of their team. I cannot say enough about all the things they taught me. Internships are a rare opportunity to taste a career. It is even more rare to find people like these who are so committed to what they do that they generously welcomed this newcomer in with open arms, taking the time to mentor and work with me.

Another unexpected teacher is Bryan Arendall. I met Bryan, a postdoctoral researcher, when I first started working with Dave and Jane Richardson in the department of biochemistry. Although I have a wonderful relationship with Bryan now, I believe that at first he thought I wasn't all that serious about learning about the field of structural biology, a subfield of biochemistry that is our lab's focus. What I found out just a few months after meeting Bryan was that he has a disability too. It showed up later in his life than mine did, and I think the shared sense of what it means to have to advocate for yourself and work hard to accommodate your disability in order to do what you want to do has strengthened our friendship. He also has taught me a great deal about how to set priorities and how to think about difficult problems. I think these skills are incredibly important. Approaching a problem with the assumption that there is some systematic way of viewing it, and that there could be innumerable interconnected issues that go along with it, is a different mindset. This is more the mindset of what people refer to as complexity theory. It is very powerful to think about things in this way and really stretches each of us to draw upon diverse information and a wide variety of perspectives when looking at a problem. Few have done more for me in terms of helping me understand those concepts than Bryan, a mild-mannered, witty, humorous and ultimately brilliant researcher who has a passion for college basketball statistics and his beloved Kentucky Wildcats.

I'm a teacher now too: Benefiting from the expertise of others over the years, and having strong mentors invest in my future, has had a profound effect on me. Not only did it change my life in all kinds of ways I could have never predicted, it also motivated me to teach teenagers and young adults who have similar disabilities. During high school and the first couple of years of college, it meant I was a counselor for children with disabilities in a structured summer program provided through the village of Manlius, New York, where I grew up.

While I was in college, my longtime teacher and friend Donna Richards got me into mentoring students who have visual impairments and attend the school district where I grew up. This is an ongoing and continuously rewarding experience for me. It is interesting to hear that some of the concerns and issues the kids face today are the same I had when I was growing up. I'm a great resource for them, because I have personal experiences in coping with a visual disability. They need to interact with a real person who has dealt with similar circumstances to theirs and has successfully gotten through high school and college. It gives them an encouraging perspective.

All of these experiences have encouraged me to take on more teaching responsibilities as time has gone on. I now work with the Duke-Durham Neighborhood Partnership in Durham, North Carolina, giving outreach demonstrations of my 3-D visualizations. The target audience is middle-school students who are learning about the basics of DNA. A few of the groups that the Neighborhood Partnership brings to the campus are specifically students who live with adversity. I'm especially grateful for the opportunity to work with these students. Having been there myself because of my disability, I feel a connection with these students, and I enjoy doing everything I can to encourage them to stay in school and create and maintain an interest in science and math.

A Runner Who Is Blind vs. a Blind Runner

From a very young age I loved soccer. I played it for years, and it was only in middle school that I gave it up. I went out for the team in the seventh grade and was among the first people who didn't make it. At the time I was convinced that I was cut because of my eyesight, but I couldn't prove it. I sort of gave up sports for a while after that, until my longtime friend Rob Logan helped change that.

In the ninth grade my oldest friend, Rob Logan, told me to join the indoor track team. There are a number of people who have tried to tell me that they were the ones who got me to join the team and start running. They may have tried, but from my memory Rob was the one who turned me into a runner.

When I started on the team I was terrible. One of my coaches was Jim Nixdorf, who was at least in his late 50s and a far better distance runner than I was. I remember, that first winter on those 20-degree Sunday mornings when we would run forest trails, just thinking that it would be an achievement if I could keep up with Mr. Nixdorf. They all thought I was nuts. Here I was one of the most out-of-shape kids, and I kept showing up every single day. By the end of the spring I had gone from running just under 6 minutes for the mile to having a breakout race where I ran two miles in 11:06 and beat my friend Rob (which he was not happy about). I ran back-to-back 5:33 miles, and that was the first time I ran under 6 minutes for the mile.

I ran my butt off the summer after my freshman year and just kept getting better. But my progress didn't happen without its fair share of stumbling blocks. During cross-country season I would have to pre-run the course one or more times and try to map out areas where I might trip over things. In one instance, at Manhattan College in the Bronx, I memorized where all the major rocks were on the course and memorized the numbers of strides I needed to take so that I could navigate it. It was well worth it: That day we set the course record for average time of five runners.*

*Author's note: The technique of using memorization to run or with other sports is something I use quite often and feel is worth emphasizing. It is a great tool for the visually impaired! I am happy to share more ways this technique can be used in many different aspects of life.

While I ran well on the cross-country course, I was better on the track. Everyone always thought I was a slow distance runner and I was determined to be a decent 400-meter and 800-meter runner. I didn't quite get my wish in the 400m, but I did improve to around

50 seconds, which I was pleased with. In the 800m I was in the 1:55 range and was able to win some races. I think what I did best in high school sports was run multiple races in a single meet. I remember one particular meet where we were trying to win the meet using our strength – distance runners – and hoping that we could sweep most of the middle-distance and long-distance events to compensate for our lack of good sprinters. That day I ran the 4x400, 4x800, open 800m and 1600m all in a two-hour time period. It was brutal, and to this day I remember my coach coming up to me after I closed the 1600m with a 60-second lap to win it. He said, "Are you tired yet?" I shook my head no, then puked. He laughed and walked away.

What is really important is that running provided me a personal challenge. It gave me an outlet for my frustrations with the rest of the world. It was something that I was able to become good at only if I put in the effort and worked hard. It also taught me discipline, commitment and courage, and trained me to work in a tight pack of teammates toward a single goal. When I was a junior I realized that I might be able to run track in college if I kept at it. This really motivated me. I wanted nothing more than to go to a Division 1 college and run track. I wanted to show all those who didn't believe in me or who used to treat me poorly that not only could I be a good student, but I could become a good athlete, all while being legally blind! Nothing they said or did would stop me.

In my senior year of high school we won almost every meet our cross-country team entered and finished the season ranked second in the country. It was great to finish off my high school racing career with some great accomplishments like that. I ran well on the track too. I was recruited at a number of Division 1 schools, and ultimately applied to and accepted an offer from Duke University. I admit that I had this overwhelming feeling of pride when I got accepted. It was as if I had vanquished the expectation that I was not smart enough, or a good enough athlete, to be successful. I was also relieved that I was going to be able to get away from the sometimes stressful and, as I saw it, unwelcoming area where I grew up. I do have fond memories of some really wonderful people there, but at the time I wanted nothing more than to get out of the town I grew up in.

Tricks of the Trade

There are many adaptive tricks I've developed over the years that I use on a regular basis. Although they may work for you, the goal of telling you about them is for you to develop a useful set of tools for yourself, so you can navigate this crazy world without losing your sense of fun, creativity, and desire to go after your goals and remain motivated.

Always allow someone the easy way out: It's understandable you may get upset with someone who has treated you poorly. It takes time and the ability to keep your cool to recognize that sometimes people just don't know any better! Explaining to them what your experience is like and allowing them a graceful exit from an embarrassing situation can help you both. There is a saying: "In the end you will always regret the severity you display more than displaying compassion and your ability to forgive." It's really hard to run into the same roadblocks repeatedly with people throughout your life and not have resentment build up over time. However, it's a good rule of thumb to assume that not only are people inherently good, but that you can help steer someone toward being better by just giving them a chance and forgiving some of their fumbling along the way. Lord knows we all want others to give us a chance too. Also, if you run into the same problem over and over again, it is in your power to figure out different strategies to get around the problem.

Know when to tell a white lie: If you are at the counter at a restaurant and can't read the menu when you are ordering takeout, it just isn't worth it to go through telling them why you are squinting at the menu. Just say you forgot your eyeglasses and pass it off as being a long day. Do it with a smile and say something like, "You know how it goes, some days you just forget them."

Some hard-line disability advocates might object to this, saying that you are denying you have a disability. But I think in some instances, it's just easier to pretend you are nearsighted so that you can quickly order some good chicken pad Thai, go home and eat dinner! I do this sometimes when I've had a really long day and am at the end of my rope. It also happens to be what I order at every Thai restaurant. Most of the time I can't read the menu and I'm pretty sure that every Thai restaurant in the United States serves pad Thai.*

Author's note: I do the same thing at restaurants that have dependable menu items. When Jeremy and I discussed this — well, argued somewhat! — we agreed in general. That said, although I agree it's sometimes necessary to just take it easy when you are emotionally exhausted and don't feel like educating some-

one about your disability, it is also important to know when it is a good time to let someone know that they could make someone else's life easier. It also gives that person a chance to do a good deed that just might make their day. These are just opinions, of course! Seldom a day goes by when someone in a restaurant or store cannot restrain from commenting, "Hey, did you forget your glasses?" I do feel this is the important opportunity to forgive that person and help them understand about visual disabilities.

Read body language: You can tell a lot from the way someone walks, talks or moves their body. Reading this kind of body language can help you compensate for not seeing facial expressions. From more than about five or 10 feet away, I can tell who someone is by their voice, the way they walk, the way their arms swing, and the shape of their body — although for the most part, bodies are starting to look like blobs to me. I've become very good at this. Some of my friends know it and even try to trick me sometimes by purposely walking differently to see if I can recognize them from a distance.

Get cool shades! I have had different pairs of Oakley, Maui Jims, Serengeti and other sunglasses over the years, although Michael Stone insists on my wearing Zeal Optics! He swears by them and is certain that he could not race or train without them! The thing about this disorder is that you get to be very sensitive to light. Well, this also means that you have a legitimate reason to wear sunglasses in all kinds of situations. I wear them when using a computer, when I'm outside, or when reading. If you're going to be wearing shades all the time, you might as well get nice ones and switch it up every once in a while to keep things fresh. I know more about sunglasses than anyone reasonably should, and I've always got a cool pair of them. I would only add one little aside on this: Wearing frames that are metal – like aluminum or titanium – is not safe in active sports because the glasses will hurt you if you bang into something, whereas plastic or carbon fiber ones will break and not hurt you.

We all know that those of us with less-than-perfect vision run into things a little bit here and there.

Author's note: There is more on lens technology in Chapter 15.

Never let anyone know you got smoked! If you have a disagreement with someone, or you come across a person who doesn't treat you well, always keep your cool. After you come across an adversarial situation, completely discard the feelings you had during it and move on. Be the positive, upbeat person you know you can be. Immediately following the encounter, don't let a soul know that it upset you. I should be clear about this. I am not promoting hiding emotions. Rather, I believe that it's important to process, but that is best done at a place and time when you can take a step back and relax in a comfortable environment to do so. Sometimes when things become hectic or too much to emotionally handle at once, I excuse myself from what I'm doing, go to a restroom or a quiet place, and close my eyes for a minute and just relax and take a few deep breaths and try to relax. Then I can come back to what I'm doing refocused and re-energized. It sounds simple, but it works.

The Blessing and Curse of Adapting

The blessing of adapting well is that people don't know you have a vision problem. It's a blessing that I can gradually let people know who I am and how I tick. Warming people up is always preferable to giving them all of it at once. The fact is that when you have a disability, your life has points of difference with others' lives. What is most often neglected in the disability community is that there are a far greater number of similarities to others that one can employ to help build a sense of comfort in an effort to move discussions forward. Focus on similarities and try to balance discussions with pointing out the exact point at which you differ. Disability advocates often teach people to fight for their rights and demand things they are being denied access to. This is important in some instances, but you can't be that forceful in every experience.

For example, in college there was a cute girl in my cell biology class. I sat in the front row because I could not see well and needed to be near the instructor so I could get notes from him. She sat up front because she was a bit of a go-getter and very academically oriented. Don't get me wrong, I cared about my academics, but after coming from a tough track practice I would be tired and some days I would have preferred to be in the back in case I started to nod off without insulting the professor! Anyway, I struck up a conversation with her one afternoon and pointed out that we were in class together and both sat up front. This is not the time to say, "I sit up front because I'm legally blind and have a genetic eye disorder." Instead, we talked about other interests we had in common. It took at least a month of sitting next to me in class before she asked me why the professor would hand me notes directly after class. Then we had a discussion about how I adapted my environment to fit my needs.

I learned a painful lesson from the same cute girl. I thought I had found someone I could talk to about things that upset me, and it felt nice to have someone who would listen. But what I failed to realize was that after a certain point, I had overburdened her with my problems. I also mistook her willingness to be my friend as potential for a romantic relationship, a common problem that is better discussed in the movie *When Harry Met Sally*!

The subtle point here is: I'm a person first, who happens to have a disability. Sure, much of my life requires that I adapt in order for it to run smoothly, and this absolutely takes a lot of effort. My visual impairment is not obvious because I adapt well, but that means I have the luxury of going a month or more before having to reveal it to someone.

Always be mindful that it can inadvertently work against you to tell someone all the details of the barriers you face each day. Building relationships of any sort must include a healthy dose of positive common ground, balanced by revealing personal concerns that others might think are burdens. People whose disabilities are more obvious than ours usually don't have this luxury. Their task is much harder, but the point is important — so much so that I'll say it again — you are a person first, and you happen to have a disability.

The curse of adapting well is a double-edged sword. The benefit is, you aren't defined by your disability. But if you're able to adapt so well that others are not immediately aware that you have a disability, you can run into another set of problems. The first is that someone may think you are hiding your disability. They may feel slighted by this when you eventually share your disability with them. Someone I know once said to me, "I wish you had told me. I'm ashamed that you didn't feel that you trusted me enough to tell me."

How receptive someone is to learning that

you have a disability is really important and incredibly difficult to judge. You will encounter people who have jarring reactions that can be destructive. There are people who might think that keeping something from them makes you weak and that you are actively denying something about yourself. There are others who might think that you have been lying to them and violated any trust you've built with them. These represent a reasonable range of responses – you can imagine why people might come to these conclusions. It becomes a curse when you are not able to help them see why their conclusions don't truly represent who you are. As soon as someone reacts this way to you, you have to seize the opportunity to correct their misperception, or you risk ruining your relationship with them. It can be incredibly frustrating, but it is not impossible to fix.

I find it helpful to balance how much I gradually reveal so that I'm not later accused of hiding anything. Try to maintain a feeling for when you want to actually have an explicit discussion with someone about your disability. Make sure that there is time for it to happen and that it is not done on a whim. If you are meeting some-one casually for coffee, this is a good time to discuss it. You just have to judge the appro-priate setting. When a child has a vision prob-lem, be sure he or she consents to informing his or her friends about the disability. The par-ents, too, should discuss it with the parents of the child's friends, but only with the consent of their visually disabled child.

It's estimated that as many as 20 percent of people in the U.S. could be classified as having a disability (as defined by the Americans with Disabilities Act). That translates into one out of every five people you randomly meet on the street! This is a conservative estimate. The actual number of disabled Americans is likely much higher than one in five. It is reasonable to believe that every American knows some-one with a disability, and also likely that most people have a family member who has a dis-ability. Since this population is so widespread, it is important to remember that other people may be more receptive than you think — you can build upon joint experiences and discuss how disabilities have affected their lives, as well as yours.

Life Is Funny Sometimes

We all can recall painfully embarrassing stories from our past. It was a great moment for me when I realized I could laugh at myself about each and every one of them.

A typically embarrassing moment is when you call out to someone in a public place and realize that not only did you "recognize" the wrong person, you even got that person's gender wrong! This happens often to people with visual disabilities, and it happens to me more and more. But the reason it happens more now is that I don't worry about embarrassing myself by mistaking someone for someone else! I call out when I think I see someone I know and just laugh at myself when I get it wrong. It's a subtle reminder that even as far as I have come, I'm not perfect. I'd rather approach that with a little humility and levity, so I laugh. In my mind, a little voice reminds me, "You're good, but you're not *that* good!"

Cultivate Inspiration

I've always tried to put myself in an environment where I can succeed. I realize now that I succeed most when I tried to cultivate inspiration. This usually happens in places where people are inspiring each other in their day-to-day actions and how they approach their lives. I also notice that for the most part, I like surrounding myself with very creative people. In order to adapt well to a visual limitation or other disability, we have to be creative in all parts of our lives. I think this is why I like creative and inspiring environments so much. They tend to be the kinds of environments that encourage and accept the adaptive approach I take to my visual impairment.

Now that I've had so many people come into

my life who encourage me to do whatever it is that I want to do, I've become addicted to going in directions that others are unwilling to go, or are incapable of going. Being a trailblazer is fun, but it isn't easy. I fall a lot and I fail more times than many people are comfortable with. What I think is a selective advantage for people with disabilities is that we're used to having roadblocks placed in front of us. So when we run into barriers to success in other parts of our lives, we have the option to take the positive approach and not overreact to problems. It's just a part of life and gets added to the list of things we'll just have to adapt to and figure out. If I could get every person with a disability to view things that way, we'd go a long way in terms of reducing people's anxieties.

Wrapping It All Up

I choose to live in an environment of creativity and inspiration, and I intentionally take a positive attitude that says barriers are just a little laundry list of things to get done. As a person who has a disability, I'm constantly faced with a world that is not designed for me. I'm so thankful that my mind and body are flexible enough to adapt to the artificial designs that society places all around us!

Author's note: I share many of Jeremy's suggestions designed to help you adapt to your disability. This is clearly manifested by the fact that I insisted on his participation with this book! If you have a loved one with a vision disability or any disability, many of the points shared are fantastic advice. However, please remember that Jeremy was aware of his condition from the start. This does not diminish his experience or what he can teach us — in fact, quite the contrary. I am simply stating that it takes time to master these skills and we must be gentle with ourselves while we are adapting to the changes we now face. I am certain he would agree with me.

chapter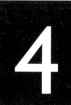

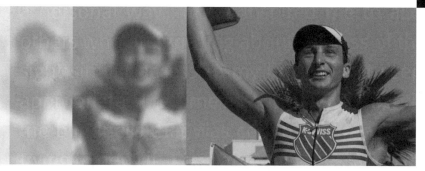

aaron scheidies

Physical therapist; elite athlete;
spokesperson for the visually challenged;
diagnosed with Stargardt's macular dystrophy

Introduction

My friendship with Aaron is based on over two years of telephone conversations that took place before we met in person, yet I feel closer to him than I do to many people with whom I have daily interactions. We have spoken hundreds of times, during both his best and his worst moments. Aaron is amongst the most genuine people I know. He is also one of the best athletes I know. Quite often the two characteristics of being good-hearted and a great athlete do not blend well, as athletes at his level tend to require a certain degree of self-involvement that leaves little room for others. This is not the case with Aaron. He is incredibly dedicated to both his work and his other life pursuits. He finds the time to balance all that he loves. I was also very excited about meeting Aaron because Stargardt's shares a common gene mutation with cone-rod dystrophy, the disease my brother and I have. For some reason, this made me feel closer to Aaron. Of course, the fact that we are both triathletes also strengthened our bond.

Aaron's story is a compilation of several conversations we have had over a few years. Some of these were over the phone and some via email. His enthusiasm for helping others is very inspiring, as are his Paralympic goals and athletic goals in general.

Aaron Scheidies' Story

Aaron's vision loss was so gradual and diffuse that he has little memory of going from sightedness to blindness, but he has vivid memories of the *effects* of his vision loss. He has vague memories of teachers noticing he had difficulty seeing the chalkboard and reading books, but he recalls that when the eye doctors could not figure out what was going on they accused him seeking attention. They sent him to neurologists and psychologists. His parents were told, "He's just playing games." When he looks back at his 10-year-old self, he laughs at the idea that anyone would think he was that devious. "I just wanted to go and play sports and get dirty and sweaty like all the other kids," he recalls.

During the sixth grade, Aaron was diagnosed with a type of macular degeneration known as Stargardt's disease. This diagnosis was a long and arduous process. After hundreds of eye appointments with many different doctors, Aaron finally was diagnosed by Paul Sieving at the University of Michigan. "Despite my disgust for the Wolverines," he joked, "I admit one good thing came out of that institution. But the [MSU] Spartans are still far superior!"

The greatest challenges in his life today are much different from those that challenged him as a kid. During his teenage years, he woke up every day with the thought that because he wasn't like everyone else, his peers would tease him, stare at him and pull pranks on him. In his middle school years, his feelings about being different and an outsider negatively affected his self-esteem. He recalls, "I let it overtake me to the point that I thought of myself as worthless." He still tried to succeed at the things that were his strengths, such as athletics, in an effort to be like everyone else.

By high school his challenges centered on becoming open to telling people that he was visually impaired and needed help. He had to learn how to adapt to new environments and people. "I also had to find the best ways to accommodate my condition. This meant I needed to learn how to cope with failure. Before I could find the best way to do things, I either ran into things or made a complete fool out of myself and then learned from those mistakes."

During his college years, Aaron's greatest challenges were learning how to adapt to his new lifestyle and identity, and being more independent. Because his college provided little in the way of physical accommodations or emotional support, Aaron learned how to advocate for himself. He says, "Some people call this lifestyle change 'getting a real job.'" Getting a real job meant that he had to refocus his career options on those that could provide real income and not be hindered by his vision condition. In Aaron's case this meant to becoming a physical therapist.

Aaron recently earned his degree in physical therapy. I asked him to share his advice on how to be successful in school.

"Getting through a visually based educational experience was not easy. There are three tips to succeeding in school that I had to learn through trial and error — it would have made things much easier if I had known them beforehand! First, you must realize that every thing in life will take a little longer even with adaptive equipment; don't let that frustrate you. I estimate that even today things take me, on average, three to four times longer than they do for fully sighted people. Secondly, it is crucial to *not* do everything on your own. Ask for help. This may mean getting a reader, a scribe, or a lab assistant who'll optimize your ability to get things done. Lastly, it is important to find your strengths and utilize them to your advantage. My strengths are my memory and my ability to communicate with others. I used these strengths to maximize my potential in school."

I'm frequently asked what drives me, and how I stay motivated and inspired to participate in all the athletic activities that I do. I asked my fellow athlete Aaron these same questions.

On motivation and drive:

"Now that I have learned to accept my vision loss, the driving force comes in the form of an intense passion to conquer life challenges. When I find myself in a challenging situation, I don't say, 'I don't think I can do this,' but rather, 'What do I have to do to get this done?' I will go to any measure or put myself through any and all hardships necessary to meet this challenge and accomplish what I set out to do. Basically, I am driven to be the best that I can be, to reach my potential."

And inspiration?

"There have been many people who've inspired and directed me on the right path. People who push themselves to the limits and overcome great odds are the ones that keep me going. I am a person who feeds off the energy of others. I am inspired by anyone who has energy, emotion and passion for life."

Sight-disabled people struggle not only with the typical challenges that everyone contends with, but also have to overcome the extra hurdle caused by our vision loss, what I call the "plus one" factor. We always have to consider the "plus one" whenever we're starting a new task, but it becomes even more challenging when we're trying to accomplish things that would be difficult even for sighted people. I asked Aaron how he defines success for himself, given the "plus one" factor.

"Success is not defined by wealth, fame or possessions. Success is defined on an individual basis. Success for me may not be success for someone else. Success is reaching your potential, accomplishing feats that push you to your mental and physical boundaries. Breaking the record for being the fastest triathlete with a disability, graduating from Michigan State University at the top of my class, and completing an Ironman triathlon were all successful moments in my life. However, if I had done just enough to make the sets in practice, graduated from college with B's and completed a sprint triathlon just to finish, then I would not feel I had been successful. For some, the latter accomplishments would be very successful, but I was born with great potential in both athletics and in academics. Success is something that you choose either to have or not have, depending on your attitude and willingness to push your limits."

Most people I interviewed suggested that their vision conditions do not define them. I personally believe that an RDD gives us an opportunity to redefine our identity and allows us to gain a new perspective. Aaron, however, says his vision condition does define him as a person.

"I am who I am because I have lost my vision. I am who I am because I have dealt with un-educated and unfair judgments placed upon me by society. I am who I am because I have learned a whole new way of life that differs from the rest of society. Although I can not say who I would be if I had full sight, I can say that I would be nothing close to the person I have become because of my visual condi-tion."

Aaron's advice to people who have vision loss, as well as to their families:

"To the family of a child diagnosed with any disability, I say, 'Don't shelter them!' To people who are blind or as close to totally blind as I am, I say, 'You've got to go out and run into things. That's the only way to learn.' To those that face the challenge of living with blindness or pro-gressively losing sight, don't expect or want to be sheltered by family or others. Not only does this make it more difficult later in life; it takes away the unbelievable excitement and joy that life can bring. The only way to love life is to live, and best way to live life is to love life.

"Many people interpret a few bad moments as meaning they have a miserable life. I have learned that smiling and laughing are a cure for all bad moments and almost all 'miserable lives.' Basically, attitude is everything!

"The thing that I want other people to know about me is that my life has not always been great, nor is it always great today. I have struggled with emotional issues about my disability, and I still do. Also, just because I have accepted my visual condition doesn't mean that I never question 'Why me?' or 'What would it be like if I didn't have this?' I still have struggles but the difference is that I have discovered my ability to be resilient."

Here are some of my thoughts about Aaron: As I said in Aaron's introduction, I have talked to him during his best and his worst. I recall a time when he was in Los Angeles finishing up the internship needed to complete his physical therapy degree. He was completely out of his element, with minimal to no help. Several times when I spoke to him, he was in tears. That said, he rallied to conquer each and every obstacle he encountered. I have better sight than Aaron and I found what he was doing intimidating and daunting, yet he completed what he set out to do. I have seen him do this in sports as well as academics.

Running right after the bike segment in a triathlon, irrespective of the duration of that bike segment, is difficult for the best of athletes. Aaron runs off the bike at such a pace that only an elite runner can guide him. He has set records for visually challenged triathletes at Olympic-distance triathlons. He beats fully sighted elite athletes, which is something beyond mere accomplishment!

Aaron's prowess is underscored by this story that involves Matt Reed, a sighted Olympian triathlete and arguably one of the world's best triathletes. I was at Matt's house recently as he packed his bags for a trip to a world cup race in London. I told him I had heard he would be guiding Aaron in an amateur race taking place right after the world cup race. I mentioned the pace that Matt would need to run with Aaron, which would not be much slower than what Matt runs off the bike. Within minutes, Matt asked me to call Aaron and tell him to find another guide – there was no way Matt would be able to run at Aaron's speed after just competing in the world cup race. As Matt's wife, Kelly, said, "It's not like Aaron is slow!" As I know Kelly and Matt well, this was a huge expression of respect for Aaron's athletic prowess!

chapter 5

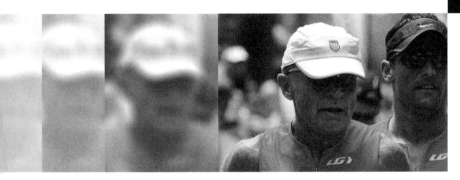

charles plaskon

Teacher; triathlete; motivational speaker;
diagnosed with macular degeneration

Introduction

I met Charlie in April of 2006, when he was 63 years old. I had just found out I would be racing in Kona that year. My parents were holding their first Foundation Fighting Blindness fundraiser in Florida, and I had asked Matt Miller of the C Different Foundation to attend and bring Charlie, who was living on Florida's west coast. Matt, Charlie's racing guide, missed the event, but thankfully Charlie and his wife, Betty, and longtime colleague Renate Frank made the event. I didn't really know any visually challenged athletes at this point and really wanted to meet Charlie.

I didn't know what to expect from an athlete who couldn't see any faces in the room, even at close distances. Someone pointed me out and he headed straight for me. He tapped me on the shoulder and promptly said, "How many miles did you run today?" That was the perfect opening statement. I immediately felt at ease with him — here we were, two poster kids for retinal degenerative diseases, attending a blindness-research fundraiser, intently talking about this morning's run rather than our vision problems. I knew I'd made a new friend. What I didn't know until very recently was that Charlie had his own story of this initial introduction, which he revealed to me almost three years later.

The fundraiser was at my parents' home, and although I knew many of the people there, I was extremely nervous. This was the first time I was no longer "Michael, Barbara and Joel's son." I was now "Michael, Joel and Barbara's visually challenged son." I could feel that those attending felt awkward as well. They really didn't know how to approach me. I could easily feel the difference. Some of those attending had known me most of my life, but they really didn't know what to say. Although I understood why it was awkward, I certainly didn't blame anyone, as I felt awkward as well. I simply hid in the back of the kitchen and stood in one spot. What I didn't know then was that when Renate recognized me and pointed Charlie in my direction, she told him, "Michael is 10 steps in front of you, but although he is surrounded by people, he is completely alone."

Renate was correct and very perceptive. There were some 150 people in the house, perhaps more, and although I was extremely grateful for their attending the function and their incredible generosity, I did feel alone. As I said, it was three years later that Charlie told me he thought about what to say for a few minutes before making his move towards me with the perfect introduction noted above. So although he made me feel at ease, saying I made a new friend doesn't really explain our special connection. Granted, I was perplexed on how he was able to find me in the room. Renate is Charlie's eyes and sometimes right and left hand. They have various systems that help Charlie navigate through many different situations. In this case, all she had to do was give Charlie my location in the kitchen and tell him precisely how many steps away I was.

You see, Charlie has a gift of helping others.

This goes well beyond just those who are visually challenged. He is a teacher to many. He shared a unique relationship with his students. Charlie took on the most challenging of kids when no one else would. He told me one story of when a frustrated student threw a chair at him that landed directly in front of where Charlie was standing. Without any hesitation, Charlie picked up the chair and brought to the student and said, "Here's the chair, but I need to know if you intended to hit me or you intentionally missed." He handed the student the chair and said, "Here is the chair. Give it another try." The student took the chair and went back to his seat. Of course Charlie's vision, albeit bad, was much better then. His eye disease is progressive, as are all the retinal degenerative diseases I discuss in this book. What Charlie has taught himself to do is *read* people without seeing them. This is what he did with me that day in my parents' house.

Over the next few years we've became good friends. I've had the pleasure of crossing the finish line with Charlie and Matt at the 2007 Florida Half Ironman, and the even greater honor of supporting Charlie in his training for the 2007 Ironman Hawaii and during the race itself. I met Charlie and Matt at the transition areas between legs (after the swim and before the bike; then after the bike and before the run) to help Charlie while Matt prepared the next leg of the race. I learned what Matt does for his athletes and I gained an insider's understanding of what all physically challenged athletes experience. That was a true gift to me!

Charlie has completed five Ironman races, and countless other triathlons and running races, with his guides. I now have a better understanding of the dedication and discipline it takes to prepare for an Ironman triathlon when you have limited-to-no vision. I am humbled when someone says to me, "I admire your discipline," because I think of Charlie and the other physically challenged athletes I know who participate in triathlons with far less sight than I have. Charlie is now developing a career as a motivational speaker and wants to return to teaching as well.

I feel that Charlie's story provides an interesting perspective because he lost his vision at a young age during a time when visual aids were few and far between. He had to adapt in a world where adapting meant "fight or flight." He clearly chose to fight! His story is compiled from conversations we've had and emails we've sent over the years. I hope you enjoy his humor and his story.

Charles Plaskon's Story

I made my untimely entry into the world in the early morning hours of September 23, 1943, in Bayonne, New Jersey, with big beautiful blue eyes. Although not known at the time, these eyes came with a degenerative macular disease called Stargardt. In the first grade, I was diagnosed with Stargardt macular degeneration. This came as a shock to my family. My father took me to numerous doctors, the majority of whom predicted a very difficult life ahead for me. There were attempts to help correct my vision with eyeglasses, but my vision cannot be corrected by eyeglasses.

Unfortunately, in the educational system of the 1940s and '50s, there were no technical aids to help with my lack of vision other than moving me closer to the blackboard. This "solution" continued throughout my primary, secondary and college years, even though there was some progress in the field of technical aids, which assisted me to a small degree. However, my vision continued to decline. Because of my limited vision, I soon realized that I could not learn in the conventional way, but in a specialized way. I had to devise other means to absorb the subject matter. At times, when a friend would tell me of difficulties with a particular subject, I shared some of the techniques I had devised for myself. I realized that my unique learning techniques could also help my sighted friends when they had difficulty understanding new subjects. I became increasingly aware that by teaching others to think about information differently, "with different eyes," they were able to "see" it. The satisfaction I felt from helping my friends inspired me to go to college to become a teacher. With the support of my family and my desire to be included in living life fully, I found ways to succeed rather than enumerating reasons to fail.

After receiving my bachelor's degree from Newark State College, I was approved for a graduate teaching assistantship at the University of Maryland in College Park. During my year there, I taught three college-level courses while working towards a master's in industrial education.

My first teaching job was at All Boys High School in Elizabeth, New Jersey. After that school year, I moved to Long Island and started teaching Industrial Education, normally called "shop" at Copiague Middle School, got married, and eventually had three children. I taught at Copiague for 31 years, off and on.

After a particularly difficult year when my vision seriously deteriorated, I decided to stop working. It was time for me to re-evaluate my life as both a visually challenged person and as a father. At this point, my two daughters were grown up enough to where they were adjusted to their own lives. However, it doesn't take your eyes to have a child, and my wife became pregnant with our third child. Life as I knew it was very difficult for me sight-wise and I wanted this new child to have a fair chance at the life he desired. I was at a point when I wanted to simply be hung up and put on a shelf. The gift of this new child forced me to re-evaluate that thought process.

I attended the Industrial School for the Blind and received education to help me cope with the increasing loss of vision. But during that year, I realized that I was not ready to sit back and let the world go by. Luckily, I was able to return to teaching at Copiague Middle School. I also decided to get a second master's degree, this time in educational administration, from Hofstra University at night while teaching during the day. Armed with this new degree, I became the adult education director for evening classes at Copiague, while continuing my regular teaching responsibilities during the day. This was 1978 and I was about to turn 35. This opened another avenue of fulfillment. Being able to reach out to young students who really needed a push added an element to my life that was incredibly rewarding. However, my needs at home dictated that a change was necessary. The environment in New York was not working out for my family. We decided that Florida would be more suitable for us all. At 55, I retired to Florida with my family.

Unfortunately, the Florida life left me feeling very unfulfilled and I needed my own change. When I was a teacher, I had always told my students to try new things, to try things that they thought might be very difficult. So I took some of my own advice and attempted running. I was 56 years old. Prior to this, I thought you took up running only if you had nothing better to do! But now I found running kept me fit and healthy and I enjoyed it. My first run was a 5K (3.1 miles), which was difficult for me as I had very little sight and was running solo. Because I was concerned I might get lost during the race, I followed a woman who was just ahead of me. After the race we talked for quite some time, and I learned that she was more than 20 years my senior at 76 years old and had run marathons! Out of the blue, she predicted that one day I would run the New York City and Boston marathons. I could tell she meant it — it wasn't an offhand, feel-good comment.

After that, I decided to double the distance by running in a 10K (6.2 miles). My first 10K run almost finished me, but I just kept practicing, getting better running shoes, and talking with people who could give me advice. It was now 2001 and I was 57 years old and took on my first half-marathon. After my first half- marathon at Disney in Orlando, I was hooked. I started to eat better, slept more, and trained to run longer distances. After running full marathons (Long Island, New York City and Boston) I remembered the woman I met at my first 5K run and her prediction. It really *had* come true!

As my comfort level at marathon distances increased, I knew I needed a new challenge. Even though my lack of vision was a limitation, I started thinking about participating in triathlons. My first sprint-distance triathlon was Escape from Fort DeSoto in DeSoto, Florida. My experience in this race taught me that swimming is my weak suit and that biking in competition is very dangerous. However, after I saw a TV program featuring Ironman Hawaii, I became completely consumed by participating in that race and decided to hitch my wagon to that star. I contacted a coach and really got serious about attaining my dream. This meant learning how to train more efficiently and following my coach's nutrition suggestions. My next triathlon was in October 2003 in Claremont, Florida. And in May 2004, I raced in my first Half Ironman at Disney in Orlando. I completed both in respectable times.

After the Disney Half Ironman, Matt Miller of

the C Different Foundation invited me to participate in the 2004 Nautica Malibu Triathlon in California. At this point my dream was to race the World Championship Hawaii Ironman. I knew that Matt's experience and resources could help me attain my dream of participating in the Ironman Hawaii. Having a relationship with Matt drew me one step closer to that dream. I had a successful triathlon in Malibu, and was able to meet the four young visually impaired athletes — in their 20s and 30s — on the C Different Ironman team.

It was at this point that Matt asked me if I wanted to be the fifth member of his C Different team. I asked him, "What could you be thinking? What could I possibly add to your youthful team of athletes?"

He replied, "It has very little to do with the athletic event itself. It has to do with life goals, life styles and life outlooks for my athletes. They are in the tunnel of life; they are choosing colleges and occupations and contemplating the rest of their lives and what will become of them in 30 or 40 years. You are not at the end of the tunnel, but you are in a section of tunnel that has much more light than the section of tunnel they are in. You have had success in college; you were employed for 32 years. In that time you married, had three children, now have three grandchildren, and you are still competing in the exact same events they are!"

I told Matt I would give him one year of my life to see where it would go — and I must tell you that has been an extremely rewarding experience. Throughout 2005 I had participated in numerous triathlon events and have had great times with Matt and the other members of the team.

When I signed on with the team, I thought C Different was about triathlons: swimming, biking and running. But over that year, I learned that C Different is much more. It is about inspiring, educating and changing the public's perception of what visually impaired people can do. During this time I also have been inspired — to return to my lifelong profession of teaching.

I have been using these events to inspire people to realize that blind and visually impaired people do have strengths and determination and can set high standards just like anyone else. There is an ever-increasing number of physically challenged individuals who do not explore life to its fullest potential. I hope to use these events to educate society and change the opinion that exists today about people with physical challenges. They can do far more than they ever dreamed possible given their physical limitation.

We must step back and remember two of the most basic and guaranteed facts that every human being is presented with. The first one is we were all born into this world, and that puts in motion our first major time constraint. The second is that we are going to leave this world and pass on to some other place that would be the other extreme of time constraint. What we do while we are on this earth is largely governed by the individual and the physical advantages or disadvantages that we are born with, as well as the level of intelligence that we are born with and, most significantly, whether external stimuli will greatly support or enhance a person's ability to develop or stifle and curtail an individual's overall worth.

Training for these races is extremely time consuming, and finding someone to train with at Charlie's specific pace — and on a matching schedule — is very unlikely. Therefore, I asked Charlie to give me an idea of how he trains for his races, as he clearly cannot have a full-time guide.

For the swimming and biking, the guide's job is relatively simple, but on the tandem bike, much more skill is required. This would be the segment where a new guide has the most difficulty, since balancing and communication are so essential. One hundred percent communication and cooperation is necessary, and this only comes after hours of practice. The majority of my training is done alone with occasional meetings with the coach, and as we get closer to a race, I would spend more time with whoever is going to be my guide, but ultimately this is less than 10 percent of my total training.

Due to the extreme distances involved in an Ironman race, I enlisted the help of a triathlon coach. I was always a reasonably good swimmer, but I needed to learn complete body coordination, and this was taught in a pool setting under close supervision by my coach. But the swim takes place in open water, which is vastly different from a pool! When I was training for the Ironman, I lived on a short canal in Florida that led to a quiet back bay. I swam in the bay for hours, two or three times a week, towing 150 feet of rope with empty bleach bottles tied to it to create drag and resistance. This really improved my technique and endurance.

For the bike, I purchased an indoor trainer and would ride in the driveway or the garage for hours. My coach educated me in proper pedaling techniques, such as using clip-in bike shoes as efficiently as possible. The rules for USA Triathlon events require sight-impaired athletes to use a tandem bike. This brings into play a whole new series of challenges. My guide and I had to learn how to clip in and start at the same time, which is a major accomplishment. After that, balancing and trying to maintain a pace of at least 20 miles per hour, while making turns and negotiating traffic, required hours of practice. We went on century rides [100-mile bike rides] to learn how to move as if we were one person, rather than two perched atop one bike! When you add the century rides to the time I spent on the trainer by myself, it adds up to a lot of riding time.

For the run, I purchased a treadmill and spent even more hours training. I would round out my week with cross-training and always scheduled one day of complete rest.

While preparing for my first Ironman, I also completed many triathlons of varying distances with the help of a guide. For the swim portion, I was tethered to my guide with a piece of surgical tubing. My guide swam next to me to keep me on course. For the run portion, I was also tethered to my guide, who would steer me through the course by pushing or pulling my right or left arm or shoulder. And for the bike segment we rode a tandem bike and that presented a unique challenge.

As we moved through traffic on the tandem bike, most of the comments I heard were positive, but inevitably there were comments like "Is that legal?" or "Who's doing the pedaling?" or "That's not fair to the rest of us!" I know at those moments those people were not seeing Charlie the athlete, but "Charlie the blind guy."

Author's note: I understand the importance of this last statement. No matter what our hobbies or professions are, the more we as visually impaired people follow our passions, the more we improve our chances of diminishing such identity descriptions. However, I personally gain much satisfaction when I pass a fully sighted person in a race with that big sign on the back of my leg that says "PC (Physically Challenged) Blind!"

chapter 6

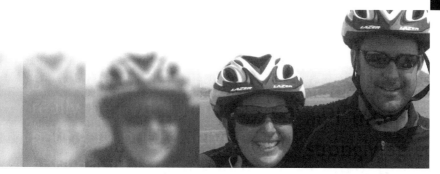

madeline cohen

Mother; federal public defender;
triathlete; rock climber; skier;
diagnosed with Usher's syndrome

At the beginning of this book I quoted my friend Madeline, who uses the powerful statement "I am *still* going blind!" as part of her fundraising efforts for FFB's VisionWalk. That provides a hint to Madeline's candid attitude about Usher's syndrome and its effect on her, and it might give you a sense of how she copes with it.

My first meeting with Madeline was a wonderful surprise that came at a crucial time in my life. My identity was evolving, from someone who "just doesn't see that well" to acknowledging that I'm visually impaired by a retinal degenerative disease that will eventually take the majority of my sight.

That was in 2006, when I had just completed racing the Hawaii Ironman as a fundraiser for the Foundation Fighting Blindness. I had received much press for that, but still knew very few people who had a retinal disease and absolutely no one of that description (other than myself!) in my hometown of Boulder, Colorado. Equally as important, I did not have any friends of my approximate age who could truly understand what I was experiencing with my vision loss. I felt isolated and lonely and *very* confused.

I was confused because although I was now receiving accolades for my accomplishments, I wasn't really doing anything new. I had been racing in Ironman as well as participating in other competitive sports activities prior to my diagnosis. The only difference was that now I knew what was causing my vision problems, and I had gone public with it by raising money for the cause of finding cures and treatments when I raced. With the diagnosis and the public acknowledgment of my disease, my seemingly normal everyday life had changed. But I had no one to share my feelings with, and really didn't feel I deserved attention for my race efforts.

This was also the year that the Foundation Fighting Blindness moved into the national spotlight with their VisionWalk. I participated in the Denver VisionWalk with Cheri Tatem, who at the time was the only local friend I knew who had a family member dealing with the effects of retinitis pigmentosa. Cheri was doing everything she could to help her mom, who has RP.

Cheri invited me to a celebratory post-Vision-Walk celebration at the home of Madeline's parents, Sara Jane and Bill Cohen. The Cohens have participated in fundraisers for years and their generosity goes well beyond raising funds for blindness research.

At the party I was introduced to Madeline, who's about my age and participates in many of the same sports as I do. I noticed that she had hearing loss as well as vision loss from Usher's syndrome, yet was confident and comfortable in a noisy room filled with strangers. I, on the other hand, was anxious and overwhelmed from being in a crowded room and not being able to distinguish people's faces. I was amazed by how easily Madeline made her way through the crowd.

When I met her family and found out how much we had in common, I wanted to become friends. I was still very much in a place of uncertainty and could not imagine how I was going to maintain a normal life or at least the life I was used to. As I chatted with Madeline she told me that she worked as a public defender. Furthermore, she was a rock climber, skier, triathlete – and the list went on. For the life of me I could not figure out how she accomplished these activities and successfully made it through school. As I mentioned, I was feeling very confused and alone about my own condition, and now I had met someone with far greater vision loss and the added challenge of hearing loss, who still was living an entirely normal life.

Here I was receiving much local press, and there was Madeline with seemingly greater physical challenges, going well beyond anything I believed I could do. If I arrived at the party confused, I left even more so, but incredibly encouraged that I now had a friend I could relate to.

It's been over two years since I first had the honor of meeting and becoming friends with Madeline, as well as her husband, mom and dad, and now her beautiful little boy. Seldom a day goes by without an invite from her mom and dad to share in a holiday or other special event.

Although she is an accomplished writer, Madeline preferred that I interview her and interpret her responses for the book. Madeline, like many others featured in *Eye Envy*, has so much to share that it's difficult to condense it all into a vignette. Also, because Madeline is so incredibly inspiring to me personally and has been a perpetual source of motivation when I need it most, I struggled with objectivity. Our initial interview took place at a local coffee shop not far from Madeline's house.

Madeline said she really did not feel worthy of being featured in this book. Instead of arguing with a trial lawyer — an argument that I would lose — I asked her, "Why?" She said she was feeling the effects of greater vision loss and it was a difficult time to discuss it. Although she wears cochlear implants[1] and can now hear somewhat better, she would love to be able to read lips. But because she has vision loss, lip reading is a challenge that is getting harder as her vision loss increases. Madeline is having a rough time coping with the changes. I am fortunate that she was open to sharing this with me. Alas, my hero is human, but still more adjusted to her condition than most. Note that as far as I know, there are fewer than 500 visually challenged practicing attorneys in the United States.

Whenever I speak with anyone who has vision loss, whether for this book or not, I ask them about their school experience. I have an expectation that those who are visually impaired experience academic challenges. It seems to be the norm, but it's not always the case.

---

1 A cochlear implant is a surgically implanted electronic device that provides a sense of sound to a person who is profoundly deaf or seriously hard of hearing.

Madeline was diagnosed with hearing loss at seven years old and then retinitis pigmentosa at 11, making it clear she had Usher's syndrome. When she said school really wasn't a problem for her, I was rather surprised, but she said all of her teachers were understanding and made concessions when necessary. She is very keen on working within her limitations. For me, this is the greatest lesson. I have made it clear that forced limitations is not a concept I take well. Knowing when to define our limitations is something we all have to live with. However, if you have a physical disability, this becomes more of a life challenge.

I told Madeline that I gave up rock climbing and skiing when my sight worsened. She admits to difficulties pursuing her athletic and recreational hobbies, but she's not willing to give them up. In rock climbing it can take some time to "approach" the actual rock face you intend to climb. The approach is essentially a hike, but the terrain can be anything from a nice trail to steep and unstable. Quite often you must cross a scree or talus field — essentially a large area of broken and wobbly rock fragments at the base of a climb or mountain cliff. She told me that some of the approaches to the climbs are her greatest challenge, but she just takes them slowly and accepts assistance when needed. She says it's disconcerting how long it takes her to get to and from the climb. I find this to be a common theme amongst most of us visually challenged outdoorsy types. We simply have to slow down a bit. It's not so horrible to trade a little speed for safety.

During our conversation, little by little, some of Madeline's hardships revealed themselves. I asked her about racing triathlons. After a bit of thought, she said she reminds herself that she can't wear cochlear implants in the water, so she swims without the ability to hear. Then she thinks about the bike portion of the race — I can see her considering what she wants to say — and she admits, "I really wish that I had something on my race uniform that says I am a visually and hearing-impaired cyclist." She says, "It scares me when the faster cyclists come flying by so closely."

The truth is, although it would make her more comfortable, athletes in a race see what they want to see and just are not expecting a visually challenged athlete to be on the racecourse, nor would they know to give her the physical space she desires. I race with a *huge* "Fight Blindness" logo on my back, but I can think of maybe four times during hundreds of races that another athlete has noticed it and responded. They ask, "What does 'Fight Blindness' mean?" I quickly explain and they usually say, "Oh, cool." And that's the end of it. It wasn't until I started racing off road that I had a friend write "PC Blind"* on the back of my calf. More athletes actually paid some attention to that.

Madeline can say what she wants about not being worthy of being in this book, but she is an inspiration to me. She just does *not* quit! I shared a racecourse with her this year in one of our hometown triathlons. After the race, she had mixed feelings about the day. The demands of her jobs as an attorney and mom leave little time to train, so she was pleased to have completed the race. But she was displeased with the lack of room people gave while passing. It's not as if she can hear them saying a polite "On your left!" Still, she participates in races and does well.

Madeline is now 37 and her vision loss is affecting her emotionally. Until now, it hasn't been so much the case. However, she's currently at a point where she's being forced to accept that she has a disability. She said, "I am going back and forth between feeling depressed and pissed off." It is conjecture on my part, but I do feel that being "pissed off" actually motivates her to move past the new limitations that are being forced upon her.

The fact that she focuses on her limitations, as well as her strengths, inspires me. For example, I can't think of anything more intimidating than standing before a packed courtroom, arguing a case in front of a judge – except doing that when you have vision and hearing problems. To me, the job seems almost impossible to do. I have shared this with Madeline, but she shrugs if off as if it's not worth mentioning, much less an inspiration to others. This speaks to that "comfort zone" I talked about in earlier chapters of this book. For Madeline, being in a courtroom is very comfortable and exciting, and it's well within her comfort zone.

I asked her, "If a 15-year-old child with Usher's syndrome were to approach you in amazement and compliment you on your career achievements, would you tell her 'It's nothing?'" Clearly Madeline doesn't give it much thought; she downplayed it even to me.

So how does she do her job? She tells each judge about her condition and says that sometimes she'll hesitate before answering the court's questions. She uses as much auditory equipment as she can, which takes out all ambient noise. But sometimes the equipment breaks down and the judges respond sympathetically.

Like me, she does not thoroughly evaluate

and utilize the new visual aids that might help her. Neither of us really understands why. It's nice to know that I'm not the only one wary of going down this path.

She says, "My job suits me." I was excited, thinking that she meant that her job is well suited to her condition, but she said that's not what she meant. She feels that although there are plenty of other career paths she could have taken, she just happens to enjoy this one. Once again, I think being an attorney *is* a fine career path for those with similar physical challenges.

The more I speak with Madeline, I realize that there is very little that she can't do, other than drive a car. She jests that she has a perfect driving record. We both laugh, as it's clear why it her driving record is perfect: She doesn't drive.

Although she says academia was not an issue for her as it was for me and so many others, she does reflect on her summer-camp days as a child. She recalls a time when she was out in the woods after dark. She had become separated from her friends and couldn't find her way back to camp. She was completely panicked, and even now she gets somewhat teary-eyed thinking about that time.

Once again, limitations enter the picture. She says that it's difficult managing the expectations of those closest to her. She doesn't want help 100 percent of the time, but wants those closest to her to know when to help and when not to. I believe this is a common theme for all of us, but I enjoyed the way she told me.

She was more specific when she said, "I think one of the hardest things about having any disability is learning how to help people help you the way you want to be helped. On the flip side, it's really hard for family members and friends to learn how to help you in a way that's useful and effective, but not demeaning or intrusive. It's a very difficult balancing act, and the answer varies for everyone, but it's important to be aware of. The best way

I know to deal with it is to be as up front as possible about what I do and do not need assistance with. I try to not take offense when people offer to help me when I don't need help or in a way that's not really useful."

This brought me to the question, "What advice would you give someone recently diagnosed with one of these diseases? What advice would you give their family?"

Madeline said, "To the newly diagnosed person: You are not disabled, and your life is not over. You may need to relearn how to do certain things, and you may need to change your day-to-day lifestyle, but you can live a full and happy life. You can be almost anything you want to be professionally (if you are not already established in your career). You can get married, you can have kids and you can travel. You can do just about anything."

To the family, she said, "Be open minded and supportive, recognize that this is a frustrating and scary condition and your family member

243

needs your help in figuring out how to adapt. Do not treat him or her as 'disabled,' and do not impose limitations on him or her through your actions, lack of support, or attitude. Work together to learn how you can be most helpful without making your family member feel disabled, and learn how you can facilitate your loved one's ability to be independent." She then said emphatically, "Advocate for your kids!"

Madeline further commented on something she's noticed about children who receive support in the early years of their diagnosis. "Kids who receive early support are able to incorporate disabilities in a neutral to positive way. For me, it was something I used to motivate me as opposed to something to fear or to hinder growth. Kids who don't receive this have greater challenges. It is essential that they receive their support from their family first."

Madeline feels inspired by those who overcome adversity and have the ability to handle adversity with grace. She credits her mom as being one of those people who are able to find humor in adverse situations. She said, "My success in life was significantly helped by my parents' getting me the services I needed."

When the coffee shop closed for the night, it was time for us to walk home. She took my arm, somewhat incredulous that *I* would be able to help *her* home. I did find it amusing that this was pretty close to an example of "the blind leading the blind." But I actually see better in the dark than I do during the daylight. That five-minute walk to her home was really special for me, as she was the one pointing out obstacles that she simply *knew* were there in an effort to protect *me,* even though I can see in those conditions better than she. It's amazing how the brain remembers such things. This is a common theme among all whom I have met who have a retinal disease.

This book features ordinary people doing extraordinary things, and Madeline is a perfect example of someone who does just that. She is very open about her fear of losing more sight and independence, yet I'm in awe of how she still gets around in the world with minimal aid. I think Madeline is extraordinary and I'm proud to call her one of my mentors.

chapter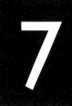

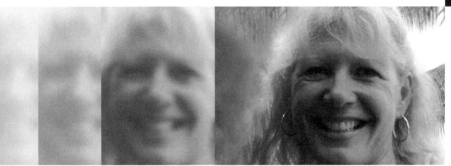

denny bettenhausen

Occupational therapy assistant; mother;
athlete; champion for helping those
with low vision; diagnosed with
Stargardt's macular dystrophy

Introduction

I met Denny by sheer luck. I was speaking at an Ironman event at Flatirons Athletic Club, the health club where I train in Boulder, Colorado. I was discussing the Race to Cure Blindness and my personal journey as an athlete who has low vision from cone-rod dystrophy. An optometrist from Fort Collins approached me and told me of a friend with a similar disease. She said her friend was an occupational therapist for people with low vision — a service I had been in great need of, but hesitated to provide for myself. I gave her my email address and she facilitated an introduction between Denny and me. After some really nice conversations, Denny told me her story, and it was so familiar it literally brought me to tears. Coincidentally, we had our diagnosis by Dr. Gerald Fishman in Chicago. I told her about *Eye Envy*, and she agreed to contribute her story to it. Furthermore, I have yet to meet someone more dedicated to helping people coping with low vision.

What can be better than a low-vision person helping other low-vision people make the most of their lives? As much as she struggled, her accomplishments far exceed the titles I gave her above! You will see my meaning as you read on. Denny is a perfect example of someone who has dealt with vision loss later in life and the challenges consistent with this loss.

Through our conversations I learned that Denny and I are both swimmers and love being around water (one has to wonder why we live in a landlocked state). Like me, she grew up in the Great Lakes area, where she was a swimmer and lifeguard and participated in aqua fitness. Denny is very close to her daughters, Melody and Harmonie. She and her daughter Harmonie took a SCUBA course together in 2003. Because things are magnified underwater, it was a whole new world underwater for Denny. SCUBA diving is now a huge part of her life, and she makes diving excursions every chance she has. She is also learning to sail, another new-found passion.

We finally met at my house, accompanied by her daughter Melody. It was a fun meeting full of levity and silly sarcasm. I showed them some of my recent artwork. Melody pointed out one of the paintings displayed on the wall that I did *not* create and she said, "I really like that *one*." I said jokingly, "Yes, that was one of my first pieces that I created, but under my *stage name*." Melody promptly said, "Wow, your work has really gone downhill," as she looked at the paintings I created. I love that kind of cheek!

Say what you want about Denny, but if nothing else she is passionate. Passionate doesn't even begin to define her sense of urgency when it comes to the subject of rehabilitation services for the visually impaired. When doctors say "There is nothing else we can do," they mean there is nothing else *they* can do. This is where the likes of Denny enter the picture. Denny was speaking about rehabilitation services for those with low vision, and I asked her how many clinics existed in the United States. Speaking from memory, she said she thought approximately 230 clinics and agencies. She then reminded me that there were well over 20 million people in the U.S. who need these services. I thought about this 20-million number, which sounded very inflated to me, since I had been using statistics of approximately 11 million. I then realized that I had only been focused on those with retinal degenerative diseases. I had been so focused on the retina that I never considered the millions with corneal and other issues, who would require therapeutic assistance simply to live as independently as possible.

I ask her how these rehabilitation services are funded. Now I have a chance to see that passionate side again. The services these clinics offer use whatever means necessary to allow anyone who is visually challenged a chance at independence. In my mind, I am thinking about the tasks I struggle with. Denny goes on to note that most people with these conditions find themselves out of work, and require such services to get themselves in a position to return to work. I think of the current unemployment situation in the U.S. Denny reminds me that a significant portion of those out of work suffer from low vision and cannot afford the services that *might* gain them at least some mobility to find work. I say "might" because many insurance companies won't reimburse for visual-rehabilitation services. Furthermore, many people don't have proper health insurance to begin with. She admits that her clinic, like many other clinics, raises scholarship funds to help those people. However, the real problem is that the clinics themselves lack the funding just to keep the lights on, and clinics such as hers are in danger of closing their doors. These clinics are nonprofit businesses and require specific funding to maintain their nonprofit status. I won't go into the details of how these funds are broken down, but the majority of their funding has to come from private donations.

It is clear to me why Denny is so passionate about this topic. Although she works very hard to advocate for these clinics, she feels vision just isn't an important enough issue for the government to listen. She really fears that with the economy being in such a horrible state, more and more clinics will be forced to close their doors. Much of the equipment that allows those who suffer from low vision a chance at independent living can be rather expensive. Some of the minor equipment I need, such as magnifiers, costs more than $1,000.

It is clear that this is just another piece of the puzzle. We need funding to research cures and treatments for these diseases; Denny strongly agrees with that statement. And we also need funding to allow people who have these diseases to enjoy life as much as possible. Cures and treatments will be nice, but what are we going to do in the meantime? Both research and rehabilitation desperately need support. Denny made a specific plea to me: to consider doing my part to assist her effort to increase awareness of these clinics, and to help raise funds to meet the needs of so many millions of people.

Please remember that Denny has Stargardt's disease, which has caused her own low-vision struggles. She is certainly doing her part to help people like me have hope for independent living.

Denny Bettenhausen's Story

The long road to getting diagnosed began when I was 18. I was mowing the lawn on a hot, humid summer day in 1977, when one of my contact lenses popped out while I was rubbing sweat out of my eyes. I tried to find the lens, but because it was green I couldn't see it in the grass. The next day I went to my optometrist, Dr. Finnegan, to get a new pair of contact lenses. He checked my vision and discovered that my prescription had changed drastically — a change that happened in less than a year from my last checkup. He had no idea why that had happened. Over subsequent months my vision continued to swiftly change for no reason that Dr. Finnegan could determine.

Dr. Finnegan researched what these changes might mean. He first referred me to a doctor at the Illinois College of Optometry, where I underwent a series of tests, and then to independent facilities when the answer still wasn't found. For five long years I met with multiple doctors and had multiple tests, which included CAT scans for pituitary tumors, tests for heavy metals, and tests that caused scratching of the cornea. Family members came in for genetic testing. More than once I went home with bandages covering my eyes. The search for an answer was painful and scary for me and my family, but Dr. Finnegan kept finding new doctors to consult. Because I was struggling with driving due to the constant vision changes, he would help me with transportation, even driving me himself if necessary. After five years of doctors and tests, I went to the University of Illinois in Chicago to see Dr. Morton Goldberg and Dr. Gerald Fishman. I was finally diagnosed with Stargardt's macular dystrophy. I was 23 years old.

Drs. Goldberg and Fishman said there was

nothing else that could be done, that I was going to be legally blind. At the time, I didn't know what this meant. No one did. I thought it meant completely blind.

Stargardt's macular dystrophy was described in 1909 by a German ophthalmologist, Karl Stargardt, after whom the disorder is named. It is an inherited condition that affects the macula, an area of the central retina, and causes loss of central vision, which is essential for reading, facial recognition and watching television or computer screens. Although there may be considerable sight loss, peripheral vision usually remains and total loss of sight is rare. It is the most frequently encountered juvenile-onset form of the group of conditions known as "macular dystrophies" or macular degeneration.

For a few years after the diagnosis, I was able to drive during the daylight hours. But when I was 29, I lost my license to drive. This was devastating for me. I became isolated, unable to ask for help and unable to persuade my family that there must be something we could do besides be helpless.

A few years later, I had an experience that convinced me I had to look outside myself for help. When my daughter Melody was about three, we lived about two miles from her day-care facility, and I took her there by bicycle. One chilly, windy autumn day when I was biking her to day care, rain started pouring down on us. Melody leaned her little head forward so that the rain wouldn't pelt her face. I could feel her forehead on my back, leaning into me, and I began to cry as we pulled into the school parking lot and saw all the other dry, warm children getting out of their parents' cars. I was grateful that the rain hid my tears.

This was my turning point. It made me look hard at my situation. I wondered how my disease was going to affect my family for the rest of our lives. We couldn't continue to ignore it. I realized I felt embarrassed about having a disability, especially one that's not obvious. Because people often wouldn't believe I had a problem, I didn't ask for help and somehow didn't believe I deserved any. People made comments like "You don't look blind," or "Yeah, I'm blind if I take my glasses off, too," or "You see better than I do!" They didn't understand that their comments reinforced the pain and anguish I felt. Each time I heard those comments I'd think, "Maybe there is something that can be done, maybe the doctors have made a mistake, because obviously I am not blind."

There is the look that people have when you tell someone you do not drive. "Really, you don't drive?" Shock and disbelief radiate from their faces. These days, what with the "green" movement, people say "Good for you!" and they don't ask about the disability, because they think you're just choosing not to use a vehicle out of principle or some environmental reason.

But before, the attitude was that I was not independent, and I was scared. People don't realize that this disease affects every single task

I do. People think that I can just correct my vision and see like they do. This left me feeling very embarrassed. I felt people thought that I wanted sympathy, when what I really wanted was understanding. But that rainy day on the bike made me realize that I need to share my experience with others. In order to get help and provide help to others, I have to explain what Stargardt's disease is and what that means to me and other people who have the disease. Once I thought of my disability differently, I was no longer embarrassed. I began a cleaning business with a sighted partner who had a car, and she would always drive us to our cleaning jobs. I also taught part time in health clubs to stay active and feel healthy.

Being active and healthy is my philosophy and my lifestyle, so it was a natural choice for me to pursue training as an occupational therapy assistant. I graduated with a degree in occupational therapy in 1993 from South Suburban Community College in Chicago. This was a feat in itself because I had felt as though I had so few options and certainly would never be able to go to school, much less graduate. Among the greatest challenges were the obstacles that my own family placed in front of me. They suggested that I accept what was happening and go on disability. They asked me, how was I going to get to campus when I couldn't drive? Where was the tuition going to come from? They couldn't imagine how I could do this without their assistance – they were afraid that I'd fail and become depressed. There was much denial and depression on my part and on my mom's part. She felt guilty about my disease, as if it were her fault I had Stargardt's. Ironically, my family's fears made me stronger in my desire to go forward in my life and figure out how to cope in spite of my vision problems.

The obstacles I encountered became personal challenges as I furthered my education. I realize now that there is a huge difference between dependence and reliance. Depending on others to get you through is helpful, but it is nothing like finding and being able to rely on your own tools to become independent.

One of the people who made that a reality for me was Katherine Eberheart, my OT instructor and mentor. She made everything accessible for me physically and mentally and encouraged me every step of the way. We are great friends to this day, and she has made a huge difference in my life and helped me on my road to independence. For that I will forever be in her debt.

Once I was accepted into the actual OTA program, Katherine sent me to Resources for Disabled Students; found a fellow student in the same program as I who took notes and enlarged them for me; taught me to record the lectures; and helped me find a car pool. She also made sure my fieldwork settings had accessible transportation available. She helped me study for boards and helped me arrange to have an alternative exam format — I was allowed to take oral exams, and when I sat for my boards, the school provided me with a reader.

During this time, I was still parenting my kids

and maintaining a full-time cleaning business. It was a challenge, for sure. My first job as an occupational therapy assistant was at St. Margaret Mercy Hospital in Hammond, Indiana. At first, I'd feel embarrassed when we would do charting (writing up patients' medical records). Co-workers would see my slow progress and say, "Maybe you need glasses." Eventually, as I became familiar with my disease, I would explain my difficulties to them. They understood, but still, there was little awareness of what the disease really meant and how it affected my performance and my self-image. When I worked with patients or other staff, I did fine, but charting and reading reports was a nightmare. I ended up taking the charts and magnifiers to a private room where I could work at my own pace in peace.

In those days I didn't have many resources available to help me cope with my diminishing field of vision. I didn't know what the challenges in my life would be, and my eye doctors never took the time to discuss it with me. I was unaware of research to find cures or treatment, and I knew of no support groups or other people who struggled with similar vision diseases. Day-to-day activities started to get more difficult to see and do. When my kids brought home their homework, I couldn't read it, and thus couldn't help them. I couldn't see the bills, nor could I read a phone book. As my kids got older, they needed rides to various activities. I always had to ask other parents to help out, but couldn't reciprocate. Someone told me about Chicago's Department of Occupational and Rehab Services (DORS), so I contacted them for services. A caseworker came to the house, interviewed me, and said I needed to learn to use a white cane. I didn't want to use a cane. I thought that because I wasn't completely blind, I didn't need that level of assistance, so I coped on my own.

I began working at the Rehabilitation Achievement Center, where I worked with people who had brain injuries. I learned more about neurological eye disorders, and interacted with many people who had double vision, blurred vision, field cuts (losing sight in one eye), and heminopsia (having only a half field of vision). I provided more vision therapy as opposed to rehabilitation, and learned about paratransit (transportation services for disabled people). I was independently getting myself door-to-door and gaining more self-confidence.

In 1995, I moved to Fort Collins, Colorado. I got a job working at the Life Care Center in Longmont, about 40 miles south of my new home. Soon after starting the job, I received a brochure about a seminar for OT practitioners and people working in vision care who would be interested in learning how to help people who have low vision. At the seminar I met Sondra Williams. She saw me sitting at a dining table, struggling to read the menu. She called me over to her table and revealed that she too had Stargardt's. Sondra taught me more about low vision and encouraged me through my very first speaking engagement, a low-vision seminar at the Congress Hotel in Chicago, where I presented with her, talking about occupational therapy for low vision.

I went to Sondra's clinics in Cañon City, Colorado, and eventually attended a four-day course in Sanibel Island, Florida, presented by Bill Mattingly and Don Fletcher. After attending this seminar I was allowed to train with caregivers and patients at Life Care Center, which was the beginning of working with patients who had previously not had their low-vision needs met. The seminar in Florida is also where I met Lila Bartmann, who changed my life! Lila really assisted my effort and became my partner to create Ensight, our low-vision center. She is also one of my closest friends.

In an effort to help my mother understand low vision, I took her to a seminar in Las Vegas to gain a better understanding of my disability. My mom took some courses at the seminar, and met other people who helped her understand what it meant to be visually impaired and how independent disabled people could be. Through these courses, she finally figured out that my vision problem was not her fault, even though it is genetic. And she realized that my disability has in some ways been re-sponsible for opening up my horizons so that I've met many more people and traveled fur-ther than I might otherwise have done.

Getting between my home and my job in-volved a 90-mile round trip every day by ex-pensive public transportation that wasn't all that convenient. When a position for a certi-fied occupational therapist assistant (COPA) in Fort Collins opened up, I applied, got the job and started a low-vision program there. Dur-ing this time I also worked for the city of Fort Collins as a water aerobics instructor. I began to serve also as the coordinator for the aqua fitness programs. The city put me on a proba-tionary period for three months because they were worried about my vision. Could I see if someone was having problems in the water? They weren't sure, but I soon proved my worth and was no longer on probation. In addition, I taught spin classes and was responsible for the fitness instructors' training.

After I was laid off from the COPA position, I

took a course to become a travel agent and started working in the field of disabled travel. I met Aida Raider, another mentor, who led me to my first Fort Collins Lions Club meeting, where I met other club members who were visually impaired. We discussed developing a clinic where people with low vision could come, meet the appropriate professionals, and learn how to cope with vision challenges. This was a lofty goal, but a goal we felt needed to be met. We believed that we could finally have a way to bring awareness about low vision to northeast Colorado communities.

By 2001, we received Lions funding for our clinic. Dr. Lou Thomas, a member of the Lions Club, was a major donor. Elderhaus, the elder day center in Fort Collins, donated space in their basement. Lila Bartmann and I volunteered for two years at no cost to our patrons. Eventually, I quit my city job and continued to volunteer at a more time-consuming pace. Then I took a job at Elderhaus, learning the finer points of successful grant writing. I worked there for one year and came up with enough funds to open an independent facility in Fort Collins. At that time, I made the decision to join Toastmasters to learn to speak confidently in public. I knew I needed to eventually go back to school, and enrolled in the online University of Phoenix in their healthcare administration program, and earned my degree. My forte is surrounding myself with excellent people, being fortunate enough to build a team who possess the skills I don't have. These people are willing to teach and believe in what we do. I have a good team. I know my weaknesses and always search to find the people that can fill those gaps.

By December 2003, Ensight Skills Center had enough funding to open our first facility in Fort Collins with a part-time paid staff, myself included. In 2006, Ensight merged with the Curtis Strong Center for Visual Rehabilitation, of Greeley, Colorado. By December 2008, we opened a satellite office in Longmont and in January of 2009, with funding support from the Fort Collins Lions Club, the Colorado Lions and the Lions Clubs International Foundation, we opened another clinic in Denver. It took three years to obtain funding for the Denver clinic, but it was worth the effort.

I am very proud of the effort we have made for our clinics. The clinics fill a very important gap between the diagnosis and the day-to-day activities life offers those who are visually challenged. It is clear that doctors can only take us so far. Very few healthcare professionals understand these visual impairments. Most just are not aware of available resources, and if they are, they don't know how to make the referrals that I have found are necessary to communicate with doctors. The day-to-day challenges for me, as for any visually impaired person, are transportation, achieving daily tasks and facing the challenges of going into dim restaurants with hard-to-read menus. As for wanting to have entertainment, going to a play or a concert where appropriate seating is limited or not available can be frustrating. Another issue is lack of awareness, as few businesses and facilities in general are set up for the challenges those with low vision have. This is why I am proud of the services we offer at our clinics, as we can make these challenges far less a problem.

Currently, I am the executive director of the Ensight Skills Center. I also am an advisor for the development of an Occupational Therapy Assistant program for Pima Medical Institute and serve on the National Accreditation Council for agencies that serve the blind and visually impaired. I am a trustee for the Fort Collins Lions Foundation and speak to thousands of people on a regular basis, giving them a chance for independence and resources, making sure people know they have options. Finally I am reaching the goal to build awareness about vision loss.

Doing this work has made me passionate about what I have to offer and has given me a mission in life. I still cannot believe that people want to hear me talk, that I am a resource for others on this level, but I stay focused and positive about my goals. I have dreamed and thought about it for so long, and now it has become a reality! Not just for me, but for so many people in our community. I am very grateful and proud to be a part of creating the Ensight Skills Center organization and all that we do. Since starting the Center in 2001, it has grown, I have grown, and I hope that the northern Colorado community has grown in understanding, awareness and support of vision loss.

eye envy

chapter **8**

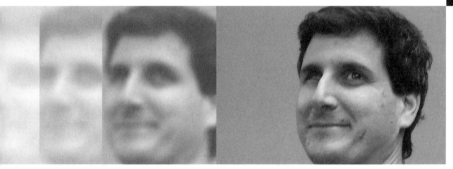

louis posen

Recording artist developer and producer;
business executive; philanthropist; father;
diagnosed with retinitis pigmentosa

Introduction

I was fortunate to meet Louis at the Foundation Fighting Blindness' Day of Science event. I found his warmth, confidence and sincerity very powerful. At the time, I was still feeling awkward around seriously visually challenged people. I didn't know what he did for a living or even why he was at the event, but I soon learned we had much in common, including our upbringing and our passion for music. The event was in San Diego, and as luck would have it, one of the bands he represents was performing the next evening. There is so much to this man of 39 years that I feel I can hardly do him justice, but he could inspire anyone to seek a sense of progress and be the best person they can. In fact, if anyone were fortunate enough to spend just a few moments with Louis, they would understand how to overcome any obstacles that might block their path.

Upon entering Louis' corporate office, you will see the following mission statement:

We create and maintain
a culture of excellence

We lead by example

We have the best interest of the
company in mind at all times

We treat our promises as commitments

We are courteous and respectful with
colleagues and outsiders at all times

We keep our work area neat
and well organized

We address problems directly
rather than speaking negatively
about them indirectly

We think about others and how what
we do and say affects others

We look inward for solutions before
looking outward

We are committed to our team goals,
not our job descriptions

We manage ourselves in order to
maximize our time

We individually strive to listen,
learn, and improve

We will go the extra mile for the team

This statement also appears on a large poster in Louis' office, and I feel it precisely describes how Louis lives his life. Granted, this is his corporate mission statement, but I am quite sure it reflects his personal philosophy. Louis is the owner and founder of a company called Hopeless Records. I am personally amused by the play on words. Hopeless Records is dedicated to helping young musicians achieve their dreams. In addition, Louis has founded several other charities. Almost all of his bands perform for a cause. The proceeds from the show we saw were dedicated to the mental health of today's youth.

Hopeless Records was founded while a young man was simultaneously going blind and finding his emerging inner vision. So, how does a young man who was diagnosed with a rare degenerative eye disease — with no treatment or cure — start a record label out of his garage in 1993 and build it into one of the most prominent independent record labels in the business?

"I did it out of a dare," Louis says, in jest and with a hint of seriousness. He adds, "Purpose, principles, people and persistence."

Today, Hopeless Records stands as one of the top 10 U.S. independent record labels. Hopeless Records recently celebrated All Time Low's release of their album *Nothing Personal*, which landed at number four on the *Billboard* Top 200, with over 63,000 albums sold in its first week. Hopeless' ground-breaking release *Waking the Fallen*, by metal giants Avenged Sevenfold, is now RIAA (Recording Industry Association of America) certified gold, with over 500,000 albums sold in the U.S. alone. The company's charitable arm, Sub City, has raised over $1.8 million for over 50 nonprofit organizations. And Hopeless Records/Sub City was recently recognized for its humanitarian work by the 110th U.S. Congress, the California Senate, the Los Angeles City Council, the National Association of Retail Merchandisers (NARM), *Billboard* magazine, *Alternative Press* and the *Los Angeles Times*, amongst many others.

In 1990, at age 19, Louis was diagnosed with retinitis pigmentosa while studying film at California State University, Northridge. Less than three years later, after being a camera assistant on various films, commercials and music videos, and directing his first video for punk's legendary NOFX, Louis started Hopeless on a dare from Orange County punk favorites Guttermouth, while filming a music video for the band.

It was just over a year after we met that I finally visited Louis in his office in Van Nuys, California. As I said earlier, I felt we had much in common, except that his vision loss is much more advanced than mine.

Louis began to notice his vision challenges at eight years old. He simply saw differences between what he saw versus what other children saw. His vision loss between the ages of eight and 19 was rather slow. He was diagnosed with RP at 19 years old, and his vision loss was very rapid after that.

Louis would be the first to warn people with compromised retinas to be very cautious with any type of medical procedure. Just after he was diagnosed, his visual acuity was approximately 20/60 in his right eye and 20/100+ in his left. He developed an abundance of ocular fluid in his right eye. Because his usual doctor at UCLA was on sabbatical, Louis was told to go to USC. He found the practice at USC to be more aggressive than what he was used to. The USC doctors convinced him that they needed to drain the fluid as part of an "easy" outpatient procedure. The result was complete vision loss in his good (right) eye. Although he had a brief adjustment in his left eye that seemed to compensate for the loss of his vision in his right eye, the cruelties of RP finally affected that eye as well.

I was terrified by this story, but Louis tells it with little regret or anger. In life, his biggest challenges stem from his own shortcomings: bad habits, insecurities and fears. He feels his eyesight problems provide their own set of material challenges, such as difficulties with transportation and reading, frustration, and sometimes embarrassing experiences that occur to those with extreme low vision. He told me, "If I can overcome the former, I would remove the obstacles of the latter." He recalls most of his relationships with his teachers and professors to be rather good. In fact, it was rare that he even bothered to tell his professors of his visual impairment. He honed his listening skills to such an extent that his are the best I've ever known. He was a film production student and, as his vision deteriorated, he turned his attention to more audio-related arts.

Louis introduced me to several of his adaptive aids. At the time I interviewed him, adaptive aids were new to me. I am just now committing to make these aids part of my life. I am currently experimenting with magnifiers and high-contrast lenses in my Zeal sunglasses that allow me to see in low light conditions that still feel bright to my eyes.

Louis defines his pre-college years as fairly normal with regard to any sight problems. He did have trouble reading for long periods of time, had some difficulty seeing the chalkboard, and had other issues that may have been related to low vision. In hindsight, he realizes that some challenges may have been due to his undiagnosed eye condition. In college, he was aware of his eyesight diagnosis, and although he did request and receive some limited assistance, he doesn't believe it had an overwhelming effect on the outcome of his overall collegiate experience. He is not suggesting that assistance for visually impaired students is unnecessary or not helpful, but rather that he limited himself by not utilizing the services available.

I asked Louis what drives him. I was sitting in the presence of a successful man who can't see the guy in front of him but seemed unaffected by it. Here's his answer:

"I am motivated by the meaning and purpose in my life, and I am inspired by so many who surround me and came before me. My wife, daughter, mom and so many others close to me help to show me how I can be a better person. I also love reading about legends such as coach John Wooden, Victor Frankel, Benjamin Franklin and Socrates, among others, who were great writers, had wisdom before their time and also could back it up with action."

"Action" is the operative word that I found particularly defines Louis!

For many of the people I've met during the process of writing *Eye Envy*, it seems that their vision impairment has redefined who they are, but I believe Louis took a different view. When I asked him whether this was true, his answer was very funny.

"Not to pull a Clinton, but it depends on how you define 'redefines you!' On one hand I don't believe any obstacle in life for anyone defines them if the definition is found in the mind, heart and soul. On the other hand, we are all affected by our obstacles, and we are who we are by how we deal with our successes and our challenges."

Louis loves quotations that hold special meaning for him, particularly those by the founding fathers of the United States. In fact, in his office is a shelf of talking dolls, including Benjamin Franklin and others from the days of the Continental Congress, which spurt out quotes from these famous men.

Benjamin Franklin was focused on making the world a better place. I recall reading that Benjamin Franklin used to awake each day saying, "What good can I do today?" I think that Louis does the very same with his day. As I wrote this, his wife was being treated for cancer, yet Louis took the time to meet with me — doing some good during a not-so-good time in his life.

It is my impression that there is little he can't do. I kept pushing him to admit that his visual impairment was a significant life challenge, but I could not get him to budge. In fact, I truly believe that his vision makes him the amazing person he is. He credits his parents for giving him a value system and for not overpowering him with limitations. He further credits them for allowing him to figure out how to adapt and overcome obstacles on his own. I asked him what advice he would give to a parent with a child recently diagnosed with a retinal disease. He said, "I would tell them to ask their child what help they want."

I had to give this some thought, as I was a little taken aback by this statement. I find it challenging to know precisely what assistance I would want and when I would want it. That thought is further complicated when I think of the various ages at which people are diagnosed with diseases that will leave them disabled. In the end, I agree with Louis that it's up to the person directly affected by a disability to seek help. However, that person might need to be nudged to define those needs.

*Author's note: This is addressed throughout the book, but children also need to know what *is possible. I mentioned earlier that I didn't even know what adaptive aids were available. So there are two issues here: knowing what's available and knowing when to ask for them.*

Louis' parents were present when he received his diagnosis, so they might have had an understanding of his issues and needs that others close to us might not. Specifically, his parents had a better understanding of his vision problems than my parents had of my vision problems because his parents witnessed his diagnosis. As I said, I have to believe Louis is correct. The person directly affected would have to figure their own pace and mobility on their own. Their loved ones can guide them, but it is up to the person who has to live with this challenge to decide what is best for them. Louis is very focused on making your own choices in life.

Louis is extremely interested in conflict resolution and wants to do his part in helping others resolve their differences. For example, a challenge that many visually challenged people try to overcome is when they find themselves impatient with others who are insensitive to the difficulties they deal with because of their vision disability. When I spoke to Louis about this, he asked me, "How do you know what *that* person's challenges are?" He also said, "Seek to understand before needing to be understood."

I think he was trying to tell me to walk in someone else's shoes before passing judgment. Also, give *listening* a fair chance — few people take the time to actually listen. I think this was his way of suggesting, "Give them a break."

I believe Louis has more empathy for those *without* vision challenges than most other low-vision people have. I often remind myself that fully sighted people just cannot relate to us. Because Louis doesn't have any vision, he isn't distracted by the sights that most people have. He is very aware of what is going on around him and in fact enjoys not having visual distractions.

Louis has learned to live with his challenges and has created a life that works very well for him. His success is defined "by achieving peace of mind, knowing you tried your best to reach your personal capacity." I believe this is something he picked up from Coach John Wooden, one of the all-time winningest basketball coaches. After hearing Louis share many of these quotes with me, I had to buy one of Coach Wooden's books!

Although I know Louis frequently quotes others, the sayings flow from him as if they are his own. It is clear to me that he lives by these beautiful words. I believe there are times that he needs such phrases to help him through the hard times. The day I spent with him at his office, his wife was at the hospital having her cancer treatments. Sadly, the day prior to our meeting, she had fallen and possibly broken a leg. She called Louis during our lunch, but the phone cut out before Louis could hear the details of her hospital visit. Her sister was looking after her, but I kept thinking how hard it must be that he could not be the one to drive her there and look after her. I know this is where Louis develops peace of mind and when personal capacity is defined. I could see how unsettled he was and how he fought being distracted by his wife's predicament. I watched his concentration flow back and forth between his concern over his wife to being present in our conversation. This is a limitation that he has accepted. Perhaps this is a lesson anyone with a challenge, be it physical or other, might accept.

There is so much more to Louis than I am capable of writing. He is very open and approachable. He mentors many young people, and has wisdom and advice to offer those affected by visual challenges, as well as to their families. I encourage anyone reading this to contact him.

Please visit his corporate website to learn more about Louis and his life endeavors: www. hopelessrecords.com.

chapter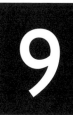

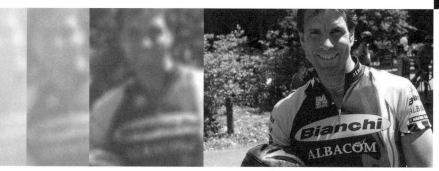

walter raineri

International tax attorney; cyclist;
competitive sailor and rower;
philanthropist; diagnosed with
retinitis pigmentosa

Introduction

I first spoke with Walter at the request of Lisa Lloyd, director of development for the San Francisco chapter of the Foundation Fighting Blindness. Walter and I are both national trustees of the Foundation. Coincidentally, Louis Posen (see Chapter 8) suggested that I speak to "Walt," as we had so much in common. Louis was speaking to Walt's passion for participating in sports. However, other than cycling, Walter and I don't really participate in the same sports. Louis tried to explain to me that Walt was a sailor. "A blind sailor?" I asked. Louis said, "I don't know how he does it either, but he does." That was all I needed, and I promptly contacted Walter.

We spoke near Walter's home in San Francisco for several hours on a beautiful afternoon in early spring. Walter is one of six siblings — four brothers and two sisters — all of whom are affected by RP. His sisters have X-linked retinitis pigmentosa, the same genetic mutation that Walter has. Although Walter has known since the age of five that he has RP, his story about coping with sight-related issues really begins when he lost 95 percent of his vision over about five months when he was 45. Prior to that time, his vision was good enough that he succeeded both in school and in his career as an international tax attorney without much struggle.

Walter exudes energy and is an eloquent speaker. He shared many stories with me, including some that provide intimate details of his experiences with RP, and I am grateful for his generosity. Walter described the progression of losing his sight as a "sack of rocks" that impeded his effort to find his "safe place." This "sack of rocks" suggests that it just weighed him down. His transformation from a "poorly functional sighted person to a highly functional blind person" allowed him to shed the rocks from his sack and lift the burden he was carrying.

As Walt is both philosophical and analytical by nature, I was interested in hearing his thoughts about "sight." Walter describes all events as experiences. I asked him what was the most meaningful experience he could share. He answered by asking me how would I define "meaningful"! He then defined it as "counter-factual thinking," saying that we are products of all our necessary bad experiences, from which we move towards a place of happiness or contentment.

We swapped many stories. I told him about my passion for cheetahs. I shared one per-sonal story that has somewhat haunted me for years. I was only 21 when I traveled to Kenya with my brother David. This was some 15 years prior to my diagnosis. I recalled an embarrassing moment when I thought I saw a cheetah and actually had our guide stop our vehicle so I could snap a photo of what was merely a tree branch and *not* a cheetah. Not wanting to miss anything, several other Range Rovers drove up to see what I was pointing at. I tried my best to maintain my pretense of see-ing something that I never really did see. I told Walt that as much as I love animals, I probably wouldn't be going on a safari any time soon, as it is such a "sighted" experience. Walt was rather sympathetic about what I felt that day in Kenya so many years ago and still feel today about this experience. We now had a definition of what a *meaningful* experience is.

As an example of meaningful experiences and an attempt to lend me some comfort, Walt shared a story about taking a South African safari after he became blind. He was with a group of sighted people who spotted a cheetah that Walter couldn't see, but by taking in the words and emotions of the group, he could imagine the scene. He also told me about "seeing" a cheetah sitting on top of a termite mound, warming herself at sunrise. Although he couldn't actually see her with his own eyes, the sighted people he was with described the scene so well, he could visualize it in his mind's eye. He says that the image he has in his head is all he needs.

Walter compares that experience with the Foundation's "Dining in the Dark" event, which is attended by sighted guests as well as those who have retinal diseases. The event begins in a well-lit room. The guests are seated and made comfortable before the dinner begins, and then the lights are turned off and the dinner commences. After about 20 minutes of dining in darkness, Walter's guests told him that they could actually "see things," even though their sense of sight was temporarily turned off. He told them that this was perfectly natural — you can visualize objects even when you cannot actually see them.

I asked Walter, "How would you advise someone recently diagnosed with a retinal degenerative disease to proceed with their life? For example, why would someone who cannot see go to the theatre, or on safari? How could people who have limited vision have meaningful experiences in these situations?"

Walter said, "The critical word here is 'meaningful.' What does it mean to have *any* experience? It's whatever gives you positive utility.

You experience it and once you do, you find out how meaningful it is to you."

Walter believes that all experiences are personal. Once you experience something, you can *then* decide how meaningful it is. For example, when going to a musical performance, some people hear the music and some people "see" it. Walter believes that when he goes to a musical event with fully sighted people, he has just as meaningful an experience as they. Each person's individual experience of the event determines what meaning and enjoyment they take from it. Those of us coping with vision loss need to value our altered perceptions, not discount them or think they're worth less because we no longer can see.

Since our meeting and many a conversation via email, Walter has become an avid rower in two-person teams. He shared with me his adventure into sailing and how he "sailed" back through the healing "waters" of losing his vision.

Walter Raineri's Story

About three years after I lost what remained of my vision, I had a couple of months when I started to feel the walls caving in on me. I had always been the guy who could do just about anything, anywhere, anytime, all the while on my cell phone talking to clients, crafting unique, innovative solutions to novel problems, as well as having a night job nourishing a handful of start-up companies. The vision loss was affecting my independence, mobility and activity. A lot of my identity was slipping away. The light at the end of the tunnel was seemingly moving farther and farther away with each passing moment.

On top of that, a long-term relationship was crumbling for the oddest reasons imaginable, and then I had a few setbacks in terms of exercise buddies. Some of the folks I normally worked out with left the Bay Area, and others who partnered with me on the tandem bicycle for endurance events were busy and cancelled our rides at the last minute. For them, these were activities that could be rescheduled or replaced with other things, but for me these activities were crucial in shoring up the caving walls. Truth be told, the eggs in my basket at that moment were few and precious, and I was protecting them to a fault.

The combination of these circumstances and setbacks left me quite down and wondering what would be next. I remember asking myself, "Should I just F 'em and F it all?" I considered cocooning in my own private world and insulating myself from all the anxiety and frustration of living in this three-dimensional world without the ability of "seeing" in three dimensions.

The turning point came when I started sailboat racing. No, not the kind that involves a joystick on a computer, or a little dinghy on a man-made pond at the local park, but open ocean and bay racing. That's right: real sailing by the really blind!

Up until June of 2008, I had never really sailed

in my life. Oh, there were those experiences out on some one's yacht or sailboat when they would tell me to do something and I did it without really knowing anything about it. My main sailing job was opening a bottle of wine and slicing cheese. But that's not real sailing. As a result, I had no expectations on my first mainstream sailing experience. This ended up being a very good thing!

The first time I went on a real sailing trip was with Captain Al Spector. My first order was to take the helm while we were at dock. I told Al that I was up for anything, but quickly added the usual disclaimer of: "I don't see very well anymore — what exactly do you want me to do with the helm?" His response rings in my ears to this very moment. "I want you to steer us out of port, and out into the bay." That was it — no hand holding, no protective barrier, nobody grabbing at me to help direct me somewhere. He didn't care if I couldn't see. This was a rare moment that was free from judgment or preconceived notions of what blind people can and cannot do. In fact, how much or little I could see seemed to be irrelevant.

To be honest, I didn't know how to respond. It had been a couple of years since I had been placed in a situation where I was asked to do something completely out of my comfort zone. None of us have any idea how many buffers are instantly created when we lose our sight. It seems that most people adopt the position that with your sight, along goes your hearing, ability to walk, ability to reason … and the next thing you know, there are invisible hands coming at you from all directions. Some hands offer truly caring support and encouragement, but others are accompanied by pitying comments — "the poor thing" — as if you're not even there. There is nothing quite like the feeling of being dragged around in the dark by well-meaning people. Or hearing the whisperers start up when you walk into a room.

Well, there I was on the boat, and a little of the punk in me came out. You know, that part of your personality that just dares to try things when others say you can't, even if you're not sure about it yourself, and you attempt it just because you don't want to be told what you can or can't do.

Being outside my comfort zone was not unfamiliar territory for me. I was used to that feeling while on the front line practicing law, and my instinct from those days told me to just go with it. Somehow, some way, I knew I would figure it out.

With only minimal instruction from Captain Al (who was initially known to me as A-1 because my computer speech synthesizer mistook the letter "l" for the number "1"), I steered us out of port and into the bay. Using a clock-face analogy (10 o'clock for a little to port, one o'clock for a little to starboard), A-1 guided me out of the docks, through Richardson Bay, down the channel, past Sausalito and into "the slot," the narrow entry to San Francisco Bay that's notoriously windy and difficult to handle. From there, I plunged into the business of learning how to sail. The learning curve was steep —

about 89 degrees! From being the helmsman to hoisting the mainsail by the mainsail halyard, trimming the mainsheet, trimming the jib, learning about the traveler placement, outhaul trimmer and vang trimmer, the experience was "out there."

Occasionally A-l would comment, "Don't fall in the water, it's damn cold and I don't want to fish you out." There was no coddling, and definitely no wine and cheese! I tried to hold a 45-degree close-reach point of sail with nothing more than the wind on my face and the noise of the rail in the water to give me course direction.

I left that first sailing experience with a renewed vigor for "getting out there." Well, "getting out there" did not take long! Within a few weeks, I was asked to join a blind sailboat racing team, and accepted without even thinking twice. The goal was to compete in the August 2008 U.S. National Blind Sailing Championships in Newport, Rhode Island, against seasoned blind racing teams from around the country. And that's what I did. Racing 10 weeks in San Francisco's "slot" is considered equal to years of experience elsewhere, so with only a summer's experience under my belt, our team headed off for Newport with me at the helm.

We did not win the fleet racing regatta in Newport, but we did compete courageously against teams with combined racing experiences of 40 years or more. The regatta in Newport elicited conflicting emotions in me. At times it was great to be there, being part of the larger event. But at other times, I was embarrassed by my lack of experience. I was so far out of my comfort zone that there were full-fledged moments of panic. I was given commands that I didn't understand but executed flawlessly, only to find out that they weren't always appropriate and had caused near collisions. Apparently, I was not the only one operating at the edge of panic.

Somehow, all this uncertainty did not bother me. It was fabulous to be engaged so deeply in an activity. All the sailing issues seemed finite, compared to the infinite set of unknown issues associated with going blind. In fact, stretching my mind to solve sailing problems of maximizing speed, understanding wind direction, perfecting sail trim, and taking advantage of tidal flows created long stretches of time in which my blindness never entered into the equation. That's the way it should be: figuring out how to deal with things as if I've always been visually impaired, rather than struggling between two worlds.

Even with me dealing with my internal struggle, the team qualified for representing the U.S.A. in the World Blind Sailing Championships in New Zealand, in the "B2" sight category. We qualified by default, in a way, because there were no other American B2 teams in the competition! The categories range from B1 to B3, with the B1 blind crew members having the least sight and the B3 blind crew members having the most. Each crew is composed of two blind and two sighted sailors. One blind sailor is designated as the helmsman and skippers the boat. The other blind sailor works the mainsheet and traveler control. One sighted sailor is the tactician, who guides the helmsman through course correction and obstacle avoidance and is only allowed to handle the self-tacking jib sheet but no other controls on the boat. The other sighted sailor is primarily a lookout and weight displacement crewmember, who's not allowed to touch any controls on the boat at all. On this team, I was the helmsman.

On the one hand, I was totally invigorated by the chance to compete with people from other countries on an international level. How many times in your life do you get such an opportunity? Hardly ever! On the other hand, it seemed like I should not be going to New Zealand with only minimal sailing experience. I mean, really, was this going to be one of those artificially created situations to simulate competition to appease the blind folk? I didn't want to be just an exhibit for sighted people to point at and say, "Look at that, the blind guy is sailing a boat!"

Still struggling with internal conflict, I headed off to New Zealand and the competition — and what a competition it was! This was no freak show. My fellow competitors could sail circles around sighted sailors, and they knew it. Most of them had at least 30 years of experience each. I worried that this could this be another one of those embarrassing situations in which the old salts would look at me and wonder why the hell I was there. Probably, I thought, as the opening ceremonies began, but: "F 'em," the little punk in me said. Somehow, I knew that my little punk was going to change my life for better or worse in the coming days!

Beyond the fact that I had no experience with the boat we were sailing, the swirling winds caused lake conditions that were nearly indecipherable to me. During the practice days, I often would become disoriented by a swirling wind that would take us off course. I kept begging for more practice time, but no one else on the team seemed to be taking my requests seriously. It seemed to me that my teammates were treating the event as if it were nothing more than a vacation activity — you know, rent a sailboat for a day and tool around the lake. How we placed in the competition seemed unimportant to them, or maybe the idea of posing a competitive threat to the more seasoned teams seemed so far out of reach that their expectations were low. Maybe just being there was an accomplishment that satisfied my teammates.

"Somehow, some way, it will get better," I kept telling myself. The drive within me to blast off to the moon was burning inside, but I lacked the tools necessary to lift off, and what burned me the most was I knew we didn't have a chance in hell.

And then the competition began.

The first two days were a disaster. I think we came in dead last in every race, often being passed by boats that started after us. After the second day of racing, I felt so embarrassed that I did not even go to the post-race BBQ that day or talk to anyone. Instead, I ran to the hotel gym and tried to center myself. Working out for five hours, I realized that in the gym there was no judgment from the weights. They couldn't care less if I could see, they only wanted to be moved around. This was nothing but cold, hard cause-and-effect relationships. And that is when it struck me – I realized that I was trying too hard, that my effort was getting in the way of my performance. I also realized that sailing is more about understanding the subtle relationships between the boat, water and wind, but the key is that you understand by *feel*, not by intellectualizing.

Have you ever had the feeling that you just need to "let go" to move forward? That's the epiphany I had during those hours in the gym.

The next day of racing was a bust. We were on the water for seven hours, but the winds were too light to start an official race. As far as I was concerned, it was the best thing that could have happened. I had seven hours to practice and internalize my feel for the boat, water and wind.

When we raced the next day, we beat the Japanese and Canadians in two races. The day after that we came in third, almost beating out the British team but missing by less than a boat length and missing second place by less than a boat length in two other races. No longer were we the token team in our division. In every race, we were right in there, mixing it up with the rest of them. It was a real tribute to our team's effort.

I started out each race day with a goal of "zero defects this race." I'd say it out loud to help me focus on "feeling" the race. As silly as that sounds, it did seem to help. I think the rest of the team thought I was losing it, but it seemed to elevate everyone's performance.

The little punk in me stood proud. In the last few races, more experienced teams were forced to jockey around us, and tried tactics to put us down — efforts reserved only for teams that presented a real threat. I wondered, how in the world did we accelerate into real competition like this? There was no way we should have even been at the championships, yet we were more than holding our own on the racecourse.

Sailing helped me tap into the little punk within me who will not be put down. The little punk had always been with me before I lost my sight. He was the source of my drive and much of my identity when I could see. It's good to know that he's still there to drive me forward.

eye envy

chapter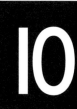

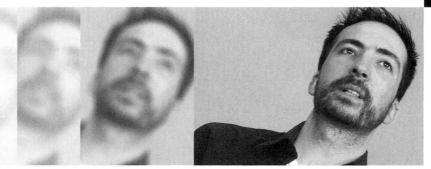

loïc burkhardt

French sound engineer
for major motion pictures; father;
diagnosed with Stargardt's disease

Introduction

For several years, I've been in close contact with Dr. Tim Schoen, a research director for the Foundation Fighting Blindness and a top champion in the field of Stargardt's disease. Because Stargardt's and cone-rod dystrophy share a common gene mutation, I am told it is likely that any new treatments for Stargardt's will also treat cone-rod dystrophy, which is the disease I have. "Dr. Tim" keeps me informed of progress in the clinical trials related to Stargardt's disease treatments, and takes an interest in my athletic endeavors and achievements. Over the years, we've become quite friendly. In fact, I met Loïc through Dr. Tim, who is Loïc's brother-in-law.

Loïc and his sister Karine, Dr. Tim's wife, have Stargardt's disease, which is the most common form of juvenile macular degeneration. The disease usually progresses much faster than cone-rod dystrophy, but has some similar effects, such as central vision loss and extreme light sensitivity.

When I first heard of Loïc, Dr. Tim told me that his brother-in-law makes the most of his life by using his hearing as a primary sense in a particularly interesting manner: Loïc is a sound engineer for motion pictures. I was beyond intrigued at this, and asked for an introduction so that I could invite him to share his thoughts and experiences with us for this book. He was gracious enough to agree, and we are fortunate indeed to have his story.

Loïc was born in 1970, and has been experiencing vision problems and sight loss since he was at least eight years old. He and his (sighted) wife were expecting a baby when I interviewed him in 2009. Clearly, they are not letting his condition affect the beauty that life offers us!

The challenge for me in telling Loïc's story is that he lives in France and his primary language is French. Most of our interviews occurred through emails. Luckily, Loïc's English is much better than my French! Although I did have to change some idioms and spellings, I have attempted to convey his story the best I could without changing the context or tone of our communications.

Loïc's Story

As much as I can recall, I didn't realize that my sight was low. In France, we have socialized care of everybody's health. A government medical doctor meets with every child to evaluate their health, and hopefully prevent, cure or take care of any special diseases. When I was about eight, I met the doctor, who believed I had a vision problem and asked to talk to my parents, but had absolutely no idea what the illness could be. My parents went with me to an ophthalmologist. He thought I had some typical problem for children of that age and suggested we needed to wear eyeglasses. I wrote "we," because my sister also had some similar problems. She's just 15 months younger than me.

A few years later, a very young ophthalmologist from our area of Valence, Thildy Normand, had the intuition that we had Stargardt's, a version of macular degeneration that affects children. She was very good, because no one else really knew about low-vision illnesses. She sent us to specialists, and that began a succession of medical tests in Lyon.

As I said, I was around eight years old and I didn't realize that I had any problems with my vision. This came later when I figured that there were things I could no longer do because of sight differences. These feelings became stronger and stronger from ages 13 to 30. And even now, slowly but surely, I lose a bit more of my vision and have to stop doing some things that I could do just a few weeks before.

Around the age of 10, I had problems with strong lights, and it was very hard for me to read anything in a brightly lit environment such as being outside, or in a classroom on a sunny day. I had to create shadows with my hands, and put the source closer to my nose to be able to read. It was hard to read the blackboard at school, and I needed to be as close as possible.

Now the symptoms are stronger. I can see larger things but without detail, and when I try to see detail, I have to move around in an effort to correct my vision enough to see. During the past three or four years, when I am tired, I see some blue shapes like blue flashes for a second. Also, objects appear to me abruptly because they are generally masked in the center of my visual field. This is very dangerous when rollerblading or bicycling, because it is challenging for me to see any obstacles. The only way to prevent it is to alter the angle of my vision in an effort to see within the healthy aspects of my visual field.

When my sister Karine and I were young, and my family realized ours was not a usual problem, the first change was that every year at the beginning of school my parents had a special meeting with my new teachers to explain that we required special arrangements. We had to sit close to the blackboard, and required larger writing on the blackboards. I was a normal kid, but after that I became something special who was treated with special care. I'm sure you can imagine what effect that has with other children at school.

As soon as we were diagnosed with Stargardt's, I had to wear sunglasses in all bright-light situations. Neither adults nor other kids could really understand why it was so important to wear sunglasses anytime, anywhere.

I had to memorize the things I would not be able to read. Reading became quickly very difficult. Thus I read as little as possible. The result is that I much later discovered the radio and culture with radio. But I also stopped reading altogether – no books for more than 20 years. Now it is late, I know, but I began using audio books, which is a revelation for me. It is very expensive, and for a sound designer it is good to let the ears take a rest, so I can't audio-read as often as I would like, but I really appreciate that medium.

Linked to that, I lost the ability to "understand" what I am reading. My reading comprehension became very much impaired. I think a part of my brain lost the capacity to comprehend long text. I can easily read and answer a usual email, but when I receive very long emails, or when I try to read a big document or a user's manual, I need to over-concentrate if I wish to understand any part of it. This process takes me a long time, a very long time.

I also slowly lost the sense of orthography (the study of spelling and how letters combine to represent sounds and form words), because of my need to stop reading and see the correct orthography of words.

My handwriting is hardly legible. I am very handicapped with the use of paper documents. I find it very difficult to read and write. I have to use my hearing faculties as my primary sense. One significant discovery was the computer, even before my vision required the zoom feature, because I could read and write legibly with a computer. I first had a PC, and soon purchased a Mac G4 and then the 24-inch iMac, because of its excellent, easy-to-use zoom feature. The Mac also lets me run my sound software. The computer and Internet are crucial for 90 percent of the things I do in my life.

My parents decided that my sister and I did not need to go into special institutions for blind or low-vision kids, so I did my studies in "normal" conditions, and I grew up with other "normal" kids. I played some sports (tennis, judo, volleyball, fencing and BMX). I wasn't especially good at them, but I think it was important to train the best I could beyond my abilities. I also had some music lessons in "normal" courses with the other kids. I also could ride a bicycle and later a little motorbike until it became dangerous for me and other people.

I don't recall these years as the best of my life, but now I think it helped prepare me for my adult life more than it would had I not had these vision problems. I'd say my worst years were from 10 to 21 with other kids of my age and also with girls (the most important subject for any teenager and older!). I later went to a psychotherapist to deal with the complexes I was suffering through.

The ability I developed to listen has been very useful to learn languages (I speak German and English), to be able to understand people I meet, and of course to work as a sound engineer.

My parents are doctors. My mother is a podiatrist, and my dad is an M.D. He was one of the best medical doctors in the area. A few months back, I visited Crest, where we lived, and I met people who told me how they missed my dad as their doctor. I think he never accepted that he was able to cure so many people, but was unable to help his son and daughter. This caused him great pain and was something he was never able to let go of and affected every aspect of his life.

I asked Loïc a number of questions about

growing up with Stargardt's disease: Did it help to have a sister who has the same problem? What was school like for you? Were your teachers helpful or problematic?

My sister and I were very close, as we are only 15 months apart in age. When I was a teenager, I must say I "hated" her for a long time. I know it wasn't rational, but I think it was linked to our vision issues.

We've been very different in many aspects of our lives, but we were tied by our vision problem. We went together to our medical exams. I was a lonely, laconic teen feeling bad and ugly, but generally doing what I was told. I was as easy on my parents as I could be, and polite at school. My sister was an attractive girl and had more fun than anything else. She was a very good person, but I think that I wasn't able to accept that and was very jealous of our differences — first of all because the "we" outweighed the "I." I remember one day my parents realized that, and promised they would try to separate my sister and me (in things that concerned our vision treatments), in an effort to let us be normal, individual persons. I think this is a typical psychological concept, but also I think it helped. Luckily our relationship today is very good.

Do you and your sister discuss your vision challenges with each another?

We don't really talk about the realities we both live with, but we do discuss new applications: a new electronic zoom, for example. We also discuss scientific news about macular degeneration. I think we have very different ways to live with our vision problems. Our attitudes differ. We manage our solutions in different ways. For instance, I early on chose an Apple computer because of the ease of use, and other advantages. She uses a PC and bought a loop system (an electronic optical aid) when it became affordable. I bought a 24-inch screen for my computer, and she uses smaller 15-inch screens and struggles with this because she doesn't want a big screen in her room. Our lives are very different and we choose very different ways to live with our vision issues.

As I said earlier, my parents met with our teachers every new school year. The result is that I could go through my "O level" equivalent (high school). I went to "normal" school and learned with the other "normal" kids. I must say that I was good at the beginning, and for that I became lazy and had some difficulties at the end because I didn't understand how to study. This is the reason why I didn't study long and brilliantly after O levels. When I went to university, I was completely lost in big rooms with too many students and I was far, very far, from the blackboard. I wanted to study physics and math, to go into very famous and select schools for studying sound. I spent most of my time trying to get my lessons from other students. I copied their notes and decrypted their handwriting. But because of this, I couldn't find time to learn and practice my exercises. I completed only one year at the Paris V University (Paris Descartes University, which concentrates on medical sciences, math and social sciences). After that I realized that I had better learn the job I wished to practice in my real professional life. I went for a training course in an animation studio called Folimage. Later, I worked there as an assistant. As a worker I could also get a professional education, so I worked and learned. I became a sound designer for Folimage and also for other studios.

After my teachers had talked with my parents, some of my teachers would really try to help. For example, they wrote larger on the blackboard and asked if I was OK. They gave me my exams with larger text. Some of them treated me as they did any other kid, some were more sensitive — maybe too much — and some others didn't believe me. I guess that's because when people see me, they cannot know that I'm "sort of blind." I don't use a white stick, I don't read Braille, I walk unassisted and do many things like sighted people, so some teachers would "test" me to see if I was a liar.

This "disbelieving" is very problematic for me. I had to prove that I could not see well. This was difficult for me because I always tried to be, and live, like others. It's still a problem for me.

The French education system is good if you have physical disabilities, because you can have extra time for exams, for example. We also had the possibility to be in a non-sunny room and have an assistant help us. However, after high school you just enter the jungle (in university) and try to survive. It is why I wanted to work as soon as possible. I must say that the university did try to help "handicapped" students with their studies. But it was the very beginning of this service, so they had a very small budget and few ways of helping. I hope the handicapped services have become better.

I first wanted to be an astronaut or an airplane pilot. "Impossible, my dear!" So then I wanted to work in cinema, as a cameraman! "Impossible, my dear. Try again!"

As I like and used to play music, I became very interested in sound. I think I'll never forget the day I saw *The Empire Strikes Back,* when I was about 10. Seeing these guys in kimonos, those big hairy puppets, with dwarves or giants in them, those metal boxes moving and almost talking — all those make-believe things became alive because of the hypercreative sound work of guys such as Ben Burt. It really shocked me. I remember I went home and took my dad's cassette recorder and replayed all the story, talking as Darth Vader or disguising my voice as a droid. I played the sounds of the laser-light sabre, the laser blasters, and the Tie and X-wing fighter ships. I think this was my first "sound" memory.

Sound gained more of my interest. When I was 14, I was given the opportunity to spend 24 hours with a sound engineer working on a project. I just sat beside him and observed this man. He was a tape cutter virtuoso, using big analog tape players and recorders. His tools were only an audio tape recorder, a white pen, scissors and some Scotch tape.

He moved a little bit of audio tape in front of the playback head, marked it, cut a piece, and pasted it somewhere else. He was playing the sounds backwards, forwards, slow and fast. I was awake the next 24 hours! I recognized some of the *Star Wars* sounds and I understood how to "play" with sounds. I'll never forget those 24 hours, because after this I always tried to imagine what the usual sounds I heard around me would sound like when slowed down, played backwards, or sped up. It burned my brain and never stopped!

I wanted to make sound for cinema, but didn't know how. I didn't know anyone who could help me find information about how to become a sound engineer. The career counselors at school are excellent for usual careers, but very bad for unique jobs. My school counselor just told me about two schools that are very challenging to be accepted in, and said I needed to be a university graduate and study math and physics. So I tried Paris Descartes University, but quit because I knew I wouldn't be able to go through university and be accepted into these great sound schools. I went to work for Folimage for the training course. I worked for free so I could learn. They gave me analog tape, a Nagra recorder, and asked me to search for sounds in their tape library (the French word is *sonothèque*). I played those sounds one by one, at any speed. They were looking for a very patient guy, able to assist them on an opera TV program. It was a very challenging job, as I had to prepare "lip-sync" animation. *[Loïc explained that lip sync means pretty much what it sounds like. Sound engineers synchronize the audio, which is recorded separately, to the animation track — word by word, precisely to each frame. I find this an amazing job for someone who doesn't see well. Apparently it* can *be done!]* I had to note frame by frame anything possible for the opera soundtrack. This included music and all voices. It was a crazy job that no others wanted to do because the opera was especially difficult. I did well and passed the tests. I did my first sound job when I was 20, as a young assistant. My job consisted of that pre-sync detection and then creating sound effects for the TV opera animation film. It was very difficult, but I wanted to do well and worked very hard. My first sound effects where absolutely awful! But I did my best and learned.

After this job, I realized there were many situations where I was not able to create the best sounds, so I went through a professional training program to learn sound theory and technique. I worked as a detector for lip-sync (because I was very good at it) and went for another two long years of professional training. This is how I learned my job: trial and error, but with great success.

In 1997, Folimage needed a sound designer for the short films they produce. They chose me and I did my first decent film. The second, *At the Ends of the Earth,* by Konstantin Bronzit, was much better! I received a lot of awards throughout the world. The sound track was very good, and we had a lot of fun making the film with Konstantin. Folimage became confident in me and I had the opportunity to practice on many different sound universes for several animation short films. My work was good. Directors were very happy with my work. They liked the fact that I didn't finish a job until it sounded perfect. People liked my work, and offered me jobs on their short films. I did many shorts films for Folimage and also for other productions.

I suit this kind of work because I enjoy the technical part, and I have a very special feeling for animation films. I love to experiment with sound universes and effects. Animation allows any idea if the sounds are right for it. We don't care about being realistic. If I want to make a footstep with a plastic spoon, nobody will object if the sound works for that situation.

Now I live in Bourg-les-Valence (in France's southeast), where Folimage is located. I work with Folimage and other production houses on animation films. I still try to alternate work with professional training sessions.

Recently I designed the sound for a feature film, *Mia et le Migou,* which was a very big and terrific experience, because the production went late finishing the images, and I had to work with other people because there wasn't enough time to finish the soundtrack by myself. I spent more of my time supervising our little team than working with my professional tools. I worked 10 hours a day, seven days a week, for five months. I couldn't sleep, I couldn't think, I couldn't *live*. It was a huge marathon. I think I was very close to burning out. I felt more tired than I ever felt before, and it's taken very long to come back from the fatigue. This experience told me I'd die for my job, which is stupid. I learned I have to watch out never to reproduce such a situation. But I did well, I can be proud of the work of this movie. It will not be my favorite film because I'd have loved to have the opportunity to tinker a little on the sounds that I had to create so quickly.

Last year I made four excellent short films, some I'm really proud about. It was a wonderful experience to have the time to design each little sound, with no stress and with excellent people.

I'd like to finish with something very important for me. Since it is very difficult for me to read, I have difficulty getting a global view. It is difficult for me to learn and evaluate by reading, so I've always been connected to friends or ex-teachers who could help me get the broader view that I can't get on my own. After that, I'm able to evaluate and explore alone. I think I've always functioned like this in my technical approach, too.

I think I chose this career because I was convinced I'd never do anything else. I think it is good to have a big wish and do my best to achieve it.

Is hearing your primary sense, given your low vision?

I think that because of my low vision I had to develop a special listening ability. I don't think I have wonderful, exceptional hearing, because when I was young I went to night-clubs, and big U2 live concerts. My ears were strongly stimulated and probably got hurt in those loud environments. With my job I often have to hear very strong and loud sounds, and I'm sure I lost some hair cells from the organ of Corti. It means I may not have such good hearing. What's important is the ability to feel and analyze sound and audio – textures. I'm sure I have developed this ability.

I think I developed the ability to pay attention to whatever I hear, and to be precise, as precise as possible, when listening. Now, when my vision is much worse, I have new sensations I never had before. This helps as long as I can see enough to continue the wonderful work I do.

But I want to say that my ears are like anybody's ears. The big thing is to get sharper and sharper precision when listening. It helps me a lot in sound design for cinema, but I am a very bad music sound mixer!

Here are some skills that I've developed because of my low vision.

Position memory locator: When I was single, I lived in a sort of messy apartment. I'm not really the king of arranging my stuff! But when I was looking for something, I was able to go directly to the place where I'd put it. Now I'm married, and my wife doesn't like a messy house, so she often moves things I just put down after arriving home from my job. It can be moved only one foot above where I had put it, but it can take me more than 45 minutes to find it. This position memory also sometimes works like an internal GPS. After I go somewhere for the first time and then try to find it again, I sometimes find the place by instinct and can't explain how. I also often get totally lost!!! (smile!)

Touch: I often don't have to use my eyes to recognize some objects I am looking for, because I can find them by touching.

How I use my vision: Because I don't see

well, I think my brain remembers other information like global shapes, attitude, ways of walking or movement. My friends are always surprised because I can come very close to them in the street and not see them, whereas I can recognize them from 30 or 50 feet away. They're often surprised when I talk about an attractive girl I noticed crossing the street ... I don't actually see the pretty girl, but I feel something from the way she walks, her confidence, maybe the sound she makes walking. My brain mixes it all and tells me "wow"!

When I was at the University of Paris, I lived on the second floor of a 12-story residence. One day the electricity broke down, so that the elevator was unusable. Every student had to walk in the dark and try to find the stairs and get out of the building to go to school. It was a huge mess, with everyone walking carefully, and many were falling down. I remember hearing some very fast steps of someone walking down the stairs and sometimes knocking into people. The person would apologize and move on. It turned out to be the blind girl who lived on the same floor as I. After she called the elevator, which didn't come, she got tired of waiting and simply went down the stairs. She didn't know the elevator wasn't working and the stairs were blocked with everyone else trying to get out of the building in the total messy blackout. We had a lot of fun talking about this upside-down situation, and laughed a lot. It was nice to be able to have something in common and to share some humor in a tricky situation.

Author's note: Loïc's story was somewhat of a turning point with my research for this book. I realized the commonality with his story and so many others that I met through the process of researching this book. Of course no two persons' experiences are the same, but as I listened to Loïc's story, it began to sound more and more familiar.

I could relate much of his experience to my own and found that we naturally compensated for many of our challenges in a similar manner. I didn't have an early diagnosis or helpful treatment from teachers, but I did have some of the same challenges with my teachers. My handwriting is also ridiculously poor, and I found that switching from a PC to a Mac was incredibly helpful with its inherent accessibility features.

In addition, Loïc's summary of hearing versus listening is also something that I could relate to. I have a passion for music. I always have, and it comes very naturally to me. I can hear tones that others can't. This makes me wonder how many other visually challenged individuals can relate to this. I also share Loïc's penchant for finding humor in our visual adversity.

chapter 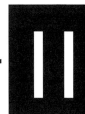 11

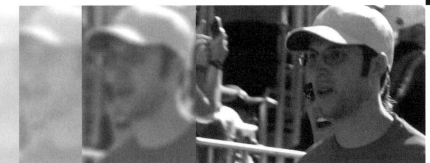

john altan kusku

High school math teacher; athlete;
diagnosed with retinitis pigmentosa

Introduction

I was introduced to John in 2008 by Mary Ann Subleski, regional director for the Midwest office of the Foundation Fighting Blindness. Mary Ann thought John and I had a lot in common, because we're both serious athletes who love to compete.

John is legally blind from retinitis pigmentosa, yet he competes at a level that surpasses the abilities of most sighted competitors. When I first met John, he was training to run in the Boston Marathon. His goal was to complete the marathon in under four hours, a time that is very respectable for fully sighted runners to accomplish. I was impressed that a legally blind runner could run a road course at that pace. I know of very few blind runners who can do this.

When I first spoke with John, I didn't yet identify myself as a visually challenged athlete, and had met few who did. Although I had received hundreds of emails from other visually challenged athletes, I really couldn't relate to them at this point. Talking to John opened me to the wider reality that I needed to learn about.

John recently graduated from Western Michigan University with a degree in mathematics. He now teaches math to high school students in Michigan. I was thrilled that he was willing to participate in this book, as he is an exceptional person who has immensely inspired me, both in his career success and in his athletic achievements.

I asked John, "When were you diagnosed, and what are your earliest memories of vision problems?"

I don't personally recall my diagnosis. According to my mother, my childhood ophthalmologist, Dr. McDonald, noticed something unusual with my retina and sent me to a retina specialist, Dr. Michael Tresse. At age five, I was officially diagnosed with rod-cone dystrophy. We later found out this was incorrect, and I now know that I have retinitis pigmentosa.

I was able to get by fairly well. At 12 years old, I used to play almost daily street-hockey games with the boys who lived two doors down. I wasn't able to follow the puck at all times, but I held my own. After a summer of being away at camp, playing goalball*, I came back home to get ready for school. I noticed the neighbors were playing hockey so I decided to run over to play. The first time the puck flew off into the grass, I was completely unable to find it. I waited for another chance. The next time the puck headed for me, I could triangulate and find it. I think that was the first time I ever knew that I could use vision by experience, but it took some effort.

John explained that goalball is a team sport designed for blind athletes. In goalball, teams of three players compete against each other to throw a ball that has bells embedded in it into the opposing team's goal. The athletes track the ball's speed and whereabouts by listening to its bells. Goalball is an official Paralympic sport.

Describe your greatest challenges.

Daily awkward interactions continue to be a challenge. For example, when I run into someone while I'm walking down the hallway, or when someone is trying to hand me something and I fumble the handoff, or I have no idea I'm being handed something. In the long run, these little flubs don't mean anything, but a ton of pebbles is still 2,000 pounds.

When I bump into someone — or almost do so, which is more common for me — I smile and say, "I'm sorry." Usually people will move on without a comment. That isn't so bad, but it isn't great. But sometimes the person I apologized to will make a rude noise, a loud exhale or a sarcastic "yeah, sure." If they do something like that and walk away immediately, I generally let it go. Those interactions actually don't make me feel that bad, because it's obvious that person has a poor attitude. Other times the person will wait to give me an opportunity to respond, or will ask me, "What are you doing?" I usually respond with

"I'm very sorry, I didn't see you" or "I'm sorry, I wasn't paying enough attention to where I was going." The latter response isn't true at all, but it is a response that most people can handle and I don't have to explain that I have a two-degree field of vision. Usually people are incredulous when I explain I'm legally blind, because I don't use a cane and I don't "look blind" — as if blind people are supposed to look a certain way and I am violating a social rule by looking "normal."

When I was 17, my friend Tyler and I had a bad experience with employees of Family Dollar in Dorr, Michigan. Tyler also has retinitis pigmentosa, and is my goalball teammate. In fact, he played for the U.S.A. goalball team in the Athens and Beijing Paralympics.

This is what happened: we went for a run and decided to pop into Family Dollar to buy a bottle of water or two. As we came up to the door, I grabbed the handle and held it open for Tyler. As he started to go through he bumped into a woman who was coming out.

He said, "Sorry, I'm blind. I didn't see you," and she responded with a rude noise. We went inside and searched around the store for some water. As I came around a corner the same woman said, "Watch out for that stack of bins. Oh, watch out for that rack," in a sarcastic, patronizing tone. When Tyler and I met up in the front of the store after concluding that they didn't sell water, the same woman said, "You don't need to lie about being blind the next time you bump into someone." I hold a grudge to this day and refuse to give Family Dollar my business.

What was school like?

School was challenging, but I worked hard and ended up with a 4.0 grade point average. I was very involved with band, and was a first-chair trumpet player and section leader. I can't really sight read. Generally I do the best I can the first few times when I read through music with an ensemble. That's usually enough to get the main ideas of the piece in my head. Then I hold the music up to my face and slowly play through the piece until I have it memorized. I don't need to memorize the entire piece, only short segments. I get to the start of a segment I have memorized; then I scan ahead to see what's next. The more I have memorized, the more fun I have with the music. If I've memorized the entire piece, then I can look at the conductor the entire time, which is wonderful. I have used this strategy my entire musical career, but I have had to rely more on memorization as my field of vision shrinks.

I marched during high school and in college at Western Michigan University. I was even a section leader at both schools. When people ask me how I stay in the formation without peripheral vision I tell them that I don't really know. I memorize where my drill tells me to be and I put myself there. I use a lot of little cheats such as keeping the bell of my trumpet positioned so it's "locked" onto the right side of the person's head in front of me. The only really tricky part in marching band was getting from the stands to the sideline and visa versa.

I had to rely on my bandmates to give me a shoulder to hold onto.

What motivates you? Is there anyone in particular who inspires you?

I am driven by a desire to do the best I can. I put a lot of time and effort into everything that I do. I specifically take being healthy very seriously. I am sure to eat fruit and vegetables each day and exercise whenever possible.

I have competed in three marathons and I play goalball competitively. Most recently I ran the Boston Marathon in 3 hours, 56 minutes. I made the U.S.A. goalball team, playing in a tournament in Lithuania and the Pan-American games in Colorado Springs.

I never run with a guide when I train. In fact I train almost exclusively on my own. I allow my mind to wander, problem-solving while I run. I only run in places I have previously traveled and know very well. That way I can focus on the things that move, such as pedestrians and cars.

I have run several 5K and 10K races without a guide, and my first marathon in Detroit was guideless. The first 4.5 miles of the Detroit Marathon are run before the sun rises, and I ran it purely by sound. I needed the sunlight to see the route, other runners and of course the aid stations where they had water and other fluid-replacement drinks and food. I kept myself between people and hoped to not run into another athlete. As there was not enough light for me to see, I didn't get any water until I crossed the bridge into Windsor and the sun was up. The best thing about that marathon is that at every aid station the volunteers are yelling "Water!" or "Gatorade!" so that the runners know which type of liquid they're offering. But what it tells me is, "There's an aid station ahead!" The aid stations tell me where I am on the route; they orient me so that I don't need a running guide to accompany me.

However, at the Boston Marathon, the volunteers do not shout out, and I would totally miss aid stations without a guide. Both times that I've run that marathon, I've had to have a guide with me. I don't use a tether, I just run beside or behind my guide depending on the crowd situation. I find it is best to just go with the flow. I have no strict rules about who follows who or which side my guide should be on. Whatever the course demands is what I do.

I ran the Detroit Marathon without a guide in 2007 in 4 hours, 3 minutes. I ran my first Boston Marathon, in 2008, in 4 hours, 44 minutes with a guide, but my guide ran out of steam. Guides can sometimes slow us down! I ran my personal best at the 2009 Boston Marathon in 3 hours, 56 minutes. My guide finished with a calm smile, while I was bawling my eyes out. No one was slowing anyone down *that* day!

Does retinitis pigmentosa defines who you are?

RP is a huge part of my life, but I don't think that it defines me. I think that my defining characteristics are my determination and goofiness. In the end I don't think that RP has very much to do with either of these traits. But it does affect how I do everything that I do.

John's advice to someone who is recently diagnosed with a retinal degenerative disease, and to their family:

Everyone has their own "stuff" to deal with. Some people have missing limbs, others have learning disabilities or are socially awkward. A visual impairment or blindness is no different. You can either focus on your disability or focus on life and learn to maximize your potential.

I really like people to meet me as a person and later on find out that I have a visual impairment. All people have a preconceived notion about who a blind person is and what he or she can and cannot do. It makes me crazy when someone defines me as being a blind person. I feel like I have to prove that I am a competent human being, and that doesn't feel very good. I much prefer to have the "So I heard you are blind — is that true?" conversation. This plan doesn't always work. For example, as a teacher I feel the need to be very up-front with my students and let them know from day one that I am legally blind. We play a few games so that everyone truly knows how much I can and cannot see.

I don't drive. I don't go to loud, dark places such as nightclubs. I don't enjoy reading print, although I love reading digitally. I don't run at night or with headphones. But other than that, I pretty much do everything that anyone else does. My advice to anyone and their families dealing with a visual impairment is to try activities even if they put you in uncomfortable situations. The best way to feel like you are living a normal life is to do normal things. I was in the marching, symphonic and jazz bands. I was highly involved in Boy Scouts, goalball, and the FFB annual auction. But as involved as I was, I wish I had done more.

Do you think that teaching is different for you than it is for sighted teachers?

If you want to have a career that you can

spend a minimum amount of time and energy on, then do not become a teacher. I think that this is good advice for anyone, but it is especially important for someone who has a visual impairment. I spend a lot of time and energy developing methods for doing things that other teachers do with ease. For example, sighted teachers can grade a math paper in about 15 seconds, but it takes me about two minutes to grade each paper. So I have students correct each other's work. This takes only a few minutes of class time and also gives an opportunity for students to understand the correct answer to each problem.

With some effort I created the perfect job for me. I have a $7,000 Promethean Board* in my classroom. The board is a 15-foot-by-8-foot interactive whiteboard mounted to the wall in my classroom, which projects whatever is on my computer screen. I also can write on the whiteboard with a special pen that's linked to software that comes with the board. I use a black background with a bold white pen. This contrast is wonderful. It makes the board very easy to read for me and for my students. The system also comes with a classroom set of personal response devices. Each device looks like a cell phone and students can answer multiple choice, numeric or text questions. I frequently set up quizzes and get immediate feedback on how students are progressing and learning. It allows me to obtain scores for students without any grading by hand.

Most teachers can glance at a student's homework page and immediately read the student's name. It usually takes me about 10 seconds to find the student's name and five more to read it. In an effort to deal with this issue, I assign each student a number (1 through 30). I ask them to write their number in the exact upper-right corner of their work. Then, after collecting their work, I have a student put their papers in numeric order, which is actually alphabetical by last name. This makes entering grades much faster. The best part of this is that it works! I am a teacher who just so happens to be visually impaired.

Author's note: The interactive whiteboard that John uses is becoming increasingly popular throughout the U.S. and Europe as a way to bring technological advances into the classroom. It's partly a way to keep kids who are used to interacting with computers interested in their lessons, but it's also a way to upgrade from the traditional blackboard. You could plan an entire lesson out and project it, bit by bit, on the interactive whiteboard and keep all the info for another year, another lesson (rather than erasing it as you do with traditional black- and whiteboards). As John shows, you can use them with clicker technology to measure and evaluate class response and who's learning and who's not, without old-fashioned tests.

Although I was introduced to John because of our athletic commonalities, what really interested me about John was his occupation as a teacher.

I originally approached John to race the Boston Marathon for the Race to Cure Blindness.

We had some difficulty connecting during that time, as he was busy with earning his degree. We only reconnected after I re-approached Mary Ann to say that I was writing a book and seeking inspiring people to feature, and that I specifically desired a visually impaired person working as a teacher. What I found interesting was that when John and I originally spoke about his racing in Boston for our cause, we really didn't connect as athletes. When I approached him in his capacity as a teacher, he really opened up!

When I think of someone standing in front of a classroom filled with fully sighted students and putting aside the fear that would accompany such a situation, I am filled with anxiety. Teaching is for the fully sighted, isn't it? At least that is what I thought until I met John.

I hope you find, as I have, that John's propensity to overcome his visual challenges and create a very healthy learning environment for his students to be a clear message that we can all overcome such obstacles.

chapter 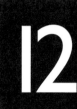12

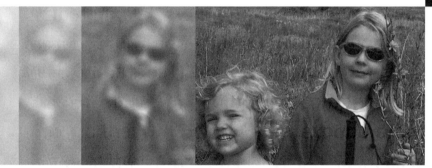

the cornell family

A parents' perspective and guide
to raising a child who has a retinal
degenerative disease

Introduction

I have spent the past few years learning about retinal diseases and meeting hundreds of affected people and their families. It became clear to me that *Eye Envy* needed a chapter from the perspective of parents. The experience that the Cornell family has had coping with LCA (Leber's congenital amaurosis) suits that need well. Since LCA can be apparent in children right from birth, families frequently confront this disease quite early on, which is what happened with the Cornells. I believe their experience and advice will help many families learn how to cope with a retinal degenerative disease of any sort, but especially those families with young children.

As with many of the people in *Eye Envy*, I met the Cornells through fortuitous circumstances. In 2006, the Foundation Fighting Blindness featured my story in their annual report, which was an enormous honor for me. Soon after the report was published, I was contacted by the Foundation, who asked if I would be willing to talk to Mike Cornell, the father of a beautiful young girl named Sela, whose story would be featured in the 2007 annual report. Allie Laban Baker from the Foundation mentioned that Sela's family also raced in triathlons as a way to raise funds for retinal research. Of course my answer was yes. Coincidentally, the Cornells lived only one town away from my parents' home. In addition, Mike's office was next to our family's office in Chicago. We also found that our business endeavors were similar. The coincidences kept piling up!

To add to the pile of coincidence, Mike worked with David Brint, who is one of FFB's directors. Of course this doesn't do David the justice he deserves, as his and his family's contribution to blindness research goes beyond words. In fact, the Brints created the first wrist bracelets used to fundraise. These bracelets were special, as they were in Braille with the added feature of glowing in the dark. The packaging featured Alan Brint, now 13 years old, who also has LCA and is another young, visually challenged person who doesn't allow his disability to be an obstacle. In fact, David told me recently that Alan has his sights on competing in a triathlon. I asked David to participate in this chapter of *Eye Envy*, as he and his wife, Betsy, are exemplary parents, but David really liked the Cornells for the chapter and modestly stepped aside.

Since meeting the Cornell family in 2006, I have become close friends with them, even helping Mike Cornell step into the Ironman triathlon world by assisting his training for Ironman Wisconsin in 2009. I am thrilled that Chrissy Cornell is still speaking to me after the intense months of training that Mike—and his family—endured. Ironman awarded Mike its prestigious Everyday Hero Award for racing his first Ironman to raise awareness and funds for retinal degenerative diseases. It makes me realize the extremes to which parents will go for their children.

I am so grateful the Cornells took the time to answer my questions and share their story to help parents and families who have a child with a retinal degenerative disease.

When did you first notice your daughter struggling?

We immediately noticed Sela's roving eye movements (nystagmus), but it wasn't until she was about two months old that we decided to press the pediatrician on the topic.

How long did the diagnosis process take?

Once the pediatrician agreed Sela's nystagmus was unusual for a child her age, he recommended we contact a neurologist. After testing via EEG technologies, the neurologist's initial comment was that Sela had a terminal brain tumor. It was without a doubt our lowest point in the process. Compounding the effects of the misdiagnosis was the neurologist's complete lack of "bedside manner." It was as though our family were in a fishbowl while doctors stopped at our exam room door to peer in and chat about Sela's purported diagnosis. From there it was an intense several weeks of MRIs. Ultimately, we were able to track down a pediatric ophthalmologist at UCLA who, after performing an ERG or electroretinogram, confirmed Sela's diagnosis of Leber's congenital amaurosis.

How were you given the news?

The pediatric ophthalmologist came into our exam room and quietly gave us the news. He briefly explained what LCA was and how it would impact Sela's vision. The initial shock was numbing, and recalling the specifics of what the doctor said is still difficult, as everything in those initial moments blurred together. To be true, we were devastated. Knowing we had a diagnosis and would not have to expose Sela to additional invasive testing was comforting, but coming to terms with the severity of her diagnosis was nearly impossible. Fortunately, as Sela's parents we were unified in an effort to support and raise our daughter as best we could. We felt strongly about providing a positive and nurturing family environment in which Sela could thrive. We also were cognizant of respecting each other's emotions and feelings about Sela's condition. This allowed us to be human, be sad, and deal with our emotions so Sela wouldn't have to.

What did the doctors tell you could be done?

They essentially told us that there was not a cure for LCA, so there wasn't anything we could really do. There wasn't a tremendous amount of support.

What help were you given?

They gave us little aid, if any at all. We took it upon ourselves to seek out resources and information about LCA. Information gleaned from our initial searches was sparse. It took months to track down an organization that knew what they were talking about. The Foundation Fighting Blindness was very helpful for this.

What is the adaptation and education process like?

Vision loss is considered a low-incidence disability, so finding services and information about how to deal with Sela's condition was an enormous undertaking. Many dead ends were hit before we started making up some ground and learning about how to help Sela. Seeking assistance through early-intervention services (provided by the government) eventually proved a great starting point. This allowed us to feel supportive and productive as Sela's parents, and helped create the basic structure that would get our family moving in a direction we felt comfortable with.

What would you want a parent to know?

Your child is your child, and they don't know any difference when it comes to vision or lack thereof. Provide your child with a caring and nurturing environment so that when they grow up they have a strong sense of themselves. We think this is the most important thing a parent can do.

Please discuss how you fundraise and why it

is important that all *parents and their extend-ed families do their part.*

When we considered fundraising options, we wanted to do something that was unique and inspirational. A triathlon ended up being the way for us to go, and it's been a blast ever since. After our first triathlon fundraiser, we had all of our athletes and supporters, friends and families attend a post-race barbeque to thank everyone for their support. It was an emotional event, and it was then we realized how fortunate we were to have so much sup-port behind Sela and our family, and at the same time how critical this group was to the success of our efforts. As individuals we can make a difference, but it's when you put all of the individual efforts together that you are able to realize the most dramatic changes.

I asked Chrissy and Mike to help me create a list of resources for parents with newly diag-nosed children in an effort to determine how you can support and advocate for your child.

U.S. Department of Education (www.usa.gov)

The information on this Web site can be limited. You might wish to contact them directly and ask the specific question you seek an answer to.

National Eye Institute (www.nei.nih.gov)

The Foundation Fighting Blindness (www.blindness.org) FFB is a very good resource for learning about the various retinal diseases.

The National Association for Parents of Children with Visual Impairments, or NAPVI (www.spedex.com/napvi)

Create a support network with other families who have children with vision disabilities. Your local FFB chapter is a good place to start.

Contact your local school for the blind, even if you are planning on having your child attend regular public school. Just for alternatives. This is of course rather personal, depending on your educational preference.

Contact your local school district to learn how to get early-intervention services for your child.

Familiarize yourself with the **IEP** (Individualized Education Program) and the **IFSP** (Individual Family Service Plan). An IEP is mandated by the Individuals with Disability Education Act (IDEA). U.S. public schools are required to develop an IEP for every student with a disability who is found to meet the federal and state requirements for special education. The IEP must be designed to provide the child with free, appropriate public education (FAPE). The IEP refers both to the educational program to be provided to a child with a disability and to the written document that describes that educational program. Key considerations in developing an IEP include assessing students in all areas related to their disability; considering access to the general curriculum; considering how the disability affects the student's learning; developing goals and objectives that make the biggest difference for the student; and ultimately choosing a placement in the least restrictive environment. An **IFSP** is similar to an IEP, but is specifically for preschool-age children, from birth to three years old.

Locate a school system/community with strong special-needs services. *This can be troublesome if you live in a community where these needs are not met. I have seen some children struggle needlessly in small towns where they just couldn't find the assistance they required.*

Seek out ophthalmologists and low-vision specialists you can work

with in the coming years. This can be a process of "trial and error." *As you read in Denny's chapter, your doctor can only take you as far as your diagnosis. They can, however, help you find alternative adaptive resources.*

Author's note: While researching where to find specific services for the blind or visual-

ly impaired, I found that most states have a Center for the Blind. This can be hidden within your state's Center for Human Services. I came across the one in Colorado when I was looking for some aid for a young adult I mentor. He was trying to take an untimed board exam to enter college and was receiving some resistance from his school. His RP was advancing quickly and he needed some outside influence. I found this group to be rather helpful.

Tips for parenting an independent and self-confident child:

Encourage your child to be capable and self-confident. Don't do for him what he can do for himself. When your child is struggling, don't rush in to rescue him — give him verbal cues that will allow him to complete a task independently.

Let your child take reasonable risks that allow her to be self-confident but don't compromise her safety.

Encourage your child to participate in most activities that her peers are participating in.

Encourage your child to advocate for himself. Encourage him to seek help when it is needed.

Don't define your child by her vision loss. It is a part of who she is, but it does not take center stage.

Author's note: Sela loves being active! She skis, rides her bike (yes, she rides a two-wheeler by herself, in controlled areas), plays outside with friends, goes to the park, reads, plays board games, watches movies, practices judo, and canoes.

The first time I met Sela, she was seven years old. We played in a park where she quickly adapted to the unfamiliar environment. I expected her to trip and bump into each and every obstacle, but this was far from the case. At first her movements were cautious, but soon she was hopping around using every piece of equipment.

This past year, I had the pleasure of having the Cornell family visit me in Boulder. It amazed me how quickly Sela adapted to my home. At first, she explored the house cautiously, especially when going up and down the unfamiliar staircase. But she soon felt completely confident in her surroundings, enough that when we heard a knock on the door, Sela rushed down the stairs to greet some of my friends who'd dropped by to visit. Although it was obvious to me that Sela compensates for her vision disability, my friends were unaware that she was not a fully sighted child until I told them. I am quite certain that even without the advances the researchers are making with LCA treatments, there will be little Sela won't be able to accomplish … I can't wait to get her into triathlon! I hope that Chrissy will still be speaking to me when there are two family members training for triathlon.

chapter 13

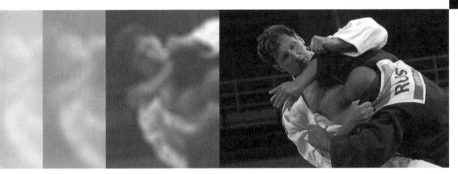

kevin szott

Olympic competitor and medal holder in judo; exercise physiologist; spokesperson for blind/visually impaired athletes; president of U.S. Association of Blind Athletes; sales manager for The Hartford Group; diagnosed with retinitis pigmentosa/macular degeneration

Introduction

As with all of the people featured in this book, it was through the most fortunate but random coincidence that I was introduced to Kevin. I was having a late-night chat with a friend and fellow athlete, Sue Huelstar, during which I told her about my vision problems. Since most people are not aware of my condition, I am used to an awkward silence when I tell them about myself. It was a relief to instead hear Sue immediately say, "This sounds very familiar! I think you have what Kevin Szott, my strength and conditioning coach at Penn State, has."

Sue gave me a little background on Kevin and, after asking her if she could track him down, I found a brief biography of him on the Web. To my surprise, Kevin was far more than "just" a strength and conditioning coach — he's also an Olympic and Paralympic competitor in wrestling, athletics, goalball and judo, who has received three gold medals, a silver and a bronze. He has an impressive bio with more accomplishments than I have ever seen in someone so affected by vision loss. I wrote and called him the very next day – I just had to meet this guy!

Kevin responded within a couple of days, and we had one of the best conversations I have had with a person with one of the inherited retinal degenerative diseases we are fighting to cure. I was in the midst of a 10-hour writing day at a local coffee shop when he reached me. I was expecting to talk for only a few minutes, but our introductory chat lasted almost two hours. This was followed by another two-hour conversation a couple of weeks later.

Kevin is a champion, plain and simple. He has so much to offer people affected by an RDD that it was a challenge to tell his story in only one chapter. For this reason, I will focus on what I believe he offers the rest of us. He is incredibly humble and modest, given his accomplishments and triumphs over blindness.

Each time we chatted, Kevin added more to his tale. For example, I was so focused on Kevin's achievements that I was surprised when he mentioned that his brother Dave is a former professional football player for the Kansas City Chiefs, Washington Redskins and New York Jets. And I was shocked to learn that Kevin was in the World Trade Center when the buildings were attacked on September 11, 2001. Thankfully he was able to safely escape, but the ordeal left him with horrific memories.

Kevin is as versatile an athlete as they come. He holds dozens of national titles in wrestling, power lifting, shot put, discus, javelin, goalball and judo for the U.S. Association of Blind Athletes, and is the second athlete ever to medal in four different sports at the Paralympic Games. He also is the first visually impaired athlete to be nationally ranked by USA Judo. During the Sydney Paralympic Games, he became the second American to win a gold medal in both Olympic or Paralympic competition. Kevin participated in the Atlanta Paralympic Games as well.

Kevin was 10 years old when he first realized he was having vision loss. Initially he was diagnosed with Stargardt's macular dystrophy, but that diagnosis was eventually revised. Kevin now knows he has an atypical form of both retinitis pigmentosa (RP) and macular degeneration. As a result, he has severe central vision loss but has maintained some peripheral vision, which is usually lost with typical RP.

Generally when I talk to people with an RDD, we follow a standard format of going through the history of their diagnosis and then the subsequent challenges of school, discussing who helped or mentored them, and how. Instead, my conversation with Kevin was more solution based. I asked him, "So, someone has this disease – what is she going to do about it?"

Kevin was very clear: No one gets through life without help! Those of us with vision challenges need a little more help, but it's up to us, as no one will or can do it for you. The choice is yours. Once you go down the road of expecting that the world owes you something, you are going down a very slippery slope!

Kevin feels role models are essential. He credits Dr. James Mastro for helping him along his path. Dr. Mastro, who holds a doctorate in physical education, has written several books that every visually challenged (and non-visually challenged) athlete should read, and holds several gold medals himself in wrestling and other sports. Jim (as Kevin calls him) helped motivate Kevin to move from wrestling to judo, as both are grappling movements. Grappling is close-contact fighting without the use of weapons. Using touch to feel the movements of an opponent is a clever way for a blind or visually challenged athlete to compete while utilizing other senses to compensate for lack of sight.

Although Kevin advocates that we learn to help ourselves, he also accepts that we do need help to cope with our loss of sight. He says that he sought psychological adaptive help during the first couple of years after his diagnosis. That said, what I find most powerful is how he defines the various paths we, as visually impaired individuals, and our families can take.

He suggests that there are three paths that we can take.

The first is the "slippery slope" of thinking that life "owes us" something to compensate for our vision loss. This path should not even be an option, but is just a downward spiral of giving in.

The other two paths he refers to as "science" and "applied."

"Science" is defined as seeking treatments and cures for retinal degeneration.

"Applied" he defines as doing what you can to help as many people as you can. In Kevin's case, he wants to help people "his way," through sports. Today, Kevin is doing just that. After serving on the board of directors for the United States Association of Blind Athletes, he is now the president. Kevin has never abandoned hope for cures, but has simply found that helping others adapt and make the most of their lives is the right path for him.

My vision loss is less than Kevin's, but is progressively becoming worse, so I asked Kevin for some advice coping with the changes I am faced with.

Here's what he told me: Things have changed, but also haven't changed. You might have to change your sport or career path. You won't be a professional football wide receiver. You have to maximize your future and seek the best help in this effort. No one has ever done anything without some help.

I then asked Kevin, "What advice would you give to the parents of a child who was just diagnosed with retinal degenerative disease?"

No hurdles, no restrictions. Parents need to learn the technology that will help their child, but don't change your parenting. Get them help by a qualified third party if necessary, but don't stop your child from being anything they want to be, and do your best to help them achieve whatever that goal might be.

I am fortunate to know several athletes who have competed in the Olympic Games, but I don't know many visually impaired athletes who have. Intrigued by Kevin's experience competing in the Paralympics, I asked him to expand on what it means to him.

My experience as a Paralympian was extremely important to who I became as a person. It gave me the chance to compete among my peer group and showed me many amazing people that were doing great things with a lot less functionality than I had. It gave me the ability to represent my country and show my support for the U.S.A. and all it represents. Lastly, competing as a visually impaired athlete is no different than any other athlete. I wanted to be the best at what I did, so I tried to find the best training, coaches and facilities I could. Then I gave it my all and competed with the best athletes in the world. No regrets and no excuses.

If you want to be the best in anything you do, the responsibility is yours. You need to set the bar high, and don't let anyone tell you that it is too high. Don't compare yourself to others, since each individual has their own set of circumstances. Seek out the best training opportunity you can and work harder than anyone else does. If you dedicate yourself in this way to being the best, then you will reach your highest potential. This may or may not result in winning the gold, but you will have achieved your maximum ability with no regrets.

These last two quotations exemplify why Kevin has achieved so much. His advice will encourage anyone to do their best, but is particularly inspirational to those of us who are coping with the results of retinal degenerative disease. I saw this firsthand when I met Kevin while he was overseeing the athletes who were headed to the 2010 Vancouver Paralympic Games. If I had not known otherwise, I would not have known he was blind. His demeanor suggested such confidence that after sharing only a few moments with him, I knew why Kevin excels at what he does, both athletically and professionally.

chapter 14

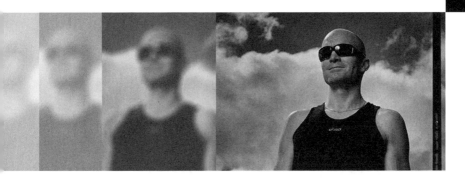

rob matthews

Father; Paralympic champion many
times over; author; diagnosed with
retinitis pigmentosa

Introduction

Rob was introduced to me by my close friend of many years Megan Gamble, who lives in Australia. Megan has had more titles than most in her very young life, one of which was editor of *Triathlon and Multi Sport Magazine*. When I embarked on this project, I of course asked her, as well as a few of her colleagues, to help me find inspiring athletes who also had one of the retinal diseases I was writing about. Through a couple of connections she found Rob.

Rob has accomplished more than I could possibly list. To start, he is one of the fastest, if not the fastest blind runner in the world. Rob falls in the same category as Erik Weihenmayer, the first blind mountaineer to summit Mount Everest, and Marla Runyan, the blind runner who competed alongside fully sighted athletes at the Sydney Olympics. Like them, Rob has written a book about his adventures and overcoming adversity, which he titled *Running Blind.* It is an amazing story that also tells how he copes with vision loss.

Rob and I have not yet met in person, but we had several wonderful conversations via email. I believe you can find and purchase his book *Running Blind* online at www.collinsbooks.com.au My friends Irene and Ray Docherty, who live in New Zealand, brought me over a copy of Rob's book, and I can't wait to read it!

Rob's Story

In my mind's eye I can still see everything. I remember clearly defined images, spectrums of colour, light and shade, but most of all I remember the face of a frightened 15-year-old staring back at me in the mirror. This is the last image I have of myself, stored away as my sight disintegrated. Like most teenagers I was scared of what lay ahead. Unlike most teenagers I had reason to be scared. I was losing my sight. Five years later, at the age of 20, I was blind.

Still, I consider myself fortunate because I have so many vivid memories from those first 20 years of my life. I can picture my sister's blond hair and her green eyes, and my dad sitting in his armchair smoking his pipe. I can recall the waves crashing against the rocks and the incoming tide gradually changing the dry, golden sand into a damp brown mass. I can see white marshmallow clouds against a mid-blue sky, and I remember the colours of the houses and the hotels on the Monopoly board, a game we played for hours on end as the rain made a mockery of another English summer. For the most part I remember living a normal, happy childhood.

I got into lots of adventures with my mates, like most young boys do, and I was your typical gawky teenager. But try as I might to fit in, my failing sight made me different, and it was something I resented at the time. I just wanted to be normal. It is ironic, really, because since I lost my sight I've rebelled against the norms of what's expected when you're blind. If someone says, "That's not something a blind man can do," then I set out to prove them wrong.

I made it my goal to be the fastest blind man in the world, and I've achieved more than I ever dreamed of on the track. I've won eight gold medals at seven Paralympic Games, set 22 world records, and was awarded the MBE for Services to Sport for the Disabled by Her Majesty the Queen. Away from running, I've driven a racecar around Brands Hatch at 80 miles per hour. I've cycled across the U.K. and Europe. I've played golf and football. I've skied and scuba dived. The way I look at it, it isn't that I'm blind, it's just that I can't see.

I inherited RP from Dad, who inherited it from his mother, who probably inherited it from her father. Most people with RP don't go totally blind until their 40s or 50s, but the rare strain of RP I inherited meant I went blind much ear-lier in life. I remember lying in bed as a young boy with the lights off, looking in the direction of the bedside table, willing myself to see it. I used to hold my hand up in front of my face, convincing myself that I could see it — surely that was a shadow, an outline . . . something . . . anything? But soon I realized it was just my imagination. I couldn't see anything in the dark.

My failing sight did nothing to help my shyness and lack of self-confidence. My efforts to blend in weren't helped by some of my teachers. At the beginning of my first summer term at school, the physical education teacher told me I wasn't allowed to participate in summer sports. I guess he felt my bad eyesight and my resultant clumsiness would make me a major liability when putting the shot, not to mention throwing the javelin. It was as good as advertising the fact that there was something wrong with me, and I remember wishing the ground would open up and swallow me.

As my sight deteriorated, I began to feel increasingly sorry for myself. I am also embarrassed to admit that I felt bitter towards my dad for passing the rogue gene on to me, for condemning me to a life of blindness. Why me?

Why should I have been cursed with losing my sight when both of my sisters had 20/20 vision? But the truth is, going blind forced me to focus. It forced me to take a good hard look at myself and challenge my own and others' preconceived notions about what a blind person could do. When I started coming to terms with my sight loss, I realized self-sympathy is no sympathy at all. Dad enjoyed a full life, helping to produce and bring up three fit, happy and healthy children. Where would we have been without him? Selfish feelings were forgotten. There was no reason I couldn't live my life to the fullest too.

And I soon realized that life can be funny, compensatory and unpredictable, all at the same time. As I learned to cope with my blindness I stumbled upon an escape, more by accident than by design. Blind people can feel isolated and alone, trapped in a world of darkness. I can't say that I've never felt isolated, but I was lucky enough to find something to fill the void. I found running.

In 1979, I was 18 and started playing goalball at college. Goalball is a game specifically designed for the blind, with three players to a side, each having to wear blindfolds to eliminate any sight advantage. The ball has bells in it and is bowled underarm. The aim is to get the ball past the opposition at the other end of a badminton-sized court into their goal. Someone once called it "knock down blind man." I was good enough at goalball to be selected for Great Britain and compete in my first Paralympic Games, which were held in the Netherlands in 1980. They should have been held in Moscow with the Olympics, but Russia at that time refused to recognize the fact that they had any physically disabled people. This was never allowed to happen again. Today every country bidding to host the Olympic Games has to make equal provision for the Paralympic Games. Goalball also took me to Indianapolis for the World Championships. This was my first time to the U.S.A. Being English, I have to say that at first I was taken aback to meet such enthusiastic people who would welcome you into their homes at the drop of a hat. I couldn't believe how different this was from home. It was here that I had my first taste of pumpkin pie — what an incredible dish that is. It's always on my "must have" list whenever I return to the U.S.A.

However, it was at the Paralympic Games that one of my room-mates, a Canadian called Jacques Pilon, changed my life without knowing it. Jacques was totally blind and won the 1500-meter running with a guide who gave him verbal instructions, along with tapping or pulling his elbow, to navigate him around the running track.

Talking to Jacques and his guide made me realize for the first time that it was possible for me to run again, despite having lost the remainder of my vision.

Two years later I was motivated, I was 21, totally blind and had found my first guide runner. We wanted to use some kind of tether to run together smoothly that wouldn't restrict our arm movement. We were breaking new ground, and we developed a new way of guide running using a rope with a hand-sized loop knotted at either end for us to hold. (This system was later adopted by the International Blind Sports Association [IBSA] as the international standard.)

Through running I felt a sense of freedom and speed I had never experienced before this time. Six months after I started running, I set my first world record over 1500 meters. Over the next six years I set another 21 world records. I'm extremely proud of the fact my world record of 4:05:11 for the 1500 remains unbeaten, as does my world record for the 800 of 1:59:90. I am the only blind person to have broken the 2-minute barrier.

Athletics gave me confidence, self-belief, friends, freedom and success, and very quickly became the most important thing in my life.

After 23 years competing for Great Britain, I wanted a change in my life. I was now 45 years of age and I had always wanted to travel for fun, not just to compete. New Zealand was one of those special places I had always wanted to go. In 2006 I went, met Sarah and moved to New Zealand, leaving behind my family and friends in England. I had met and fallen in love with a "kiwi" girl and was ready to start a new life. I was soon to become a father for the first time. Sarah and I always knew that any child of ours would have a 50/50 chance of inheriting RP, but indications to date show that our two-year-old son, Thomas, has normal eyesight and good night vision and doesn't appear to have inherited the rogue gene that causes RP.

My new life Down Under opened up the opportunity to compete at triathlons and in tandem cycling. This was something I had always wanted to do. I was selected to compete for New Zealand in the World Paralympic Triathlon Championships in Australia in September 2009 and won the silver medal. First place was taken by the U.S.A. The triathlon will not be in the 2012 Paralympic Games in London, but I am determined to make it to what will be my eighth Paralympic Games, this time representing New Zealand in road cycling. That's not my only ambition, my sights are set on running the Marathon des Sables, which is a 160-mile ultra-marathon through the Sahara Desert, and also in completing a 400-mile ski/run to the North Pole. These races will take me from plus 110 degrees to minus 10 degrees.

I truly believe that anything is possible if you set your mind to it. Being blind is not a limitation. Why settle for ordinary life when it can be extraordinary?

chapter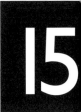

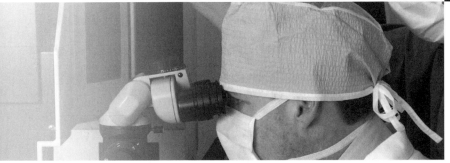

science and hope!

Learning About Retinal
Degenerative Diseases

After I was diagnosed with cone-rod dystrophy, I decided to learn about the disease and what research was being done that might someday treat it — or better yet, cure it. I heard about how gene mutations affect retinal pigment epithelial cells (RPEs) and photoreceptor cells (PCs), but this was just jargon to me, as it may be to you. So over the past few years, I have spent lots of time and energy learning about the human eye and how genetic mutations can cause retinal degenerative diseases, and in this chapter I share that knowledge with you.

I believe that everyone who has a retinal degenerative disease, or is a family member or close friend of a person with an RDD, should learn about the structure of the human eye and some basics about genetics so that you:

- understand how retinal diseases affect the eye, and become familiar with "your" retinal disease;

- understand your eye doctors and effectively communicate with them;

- are able to read about new research with-out having a brain cramp;

- can teach others about your RDD and help them understand how it affects you; and

- support new research for cures and treat-ments, because you realize that break-throughs are imminent if research is ade-quately funded.

Basic Structure of the Human Eye

The human eye is a complex organ. Its many parts work together to detect light, and con-vert it into electrical impulses that connect to the optic nerve, which is part of our brain. The retina and brain interpret the electrical im-pulses to create an image, which is what we usually mean when we talk about "sight" or "vision."

The major elements of the eye that are proba-bly best for you to learn about are the cornea, aqueous humor, iris, pupil, lens, vitreous humor, retina, macula, choroid and sclera, and the optic nerve. I *did* try to find a cool, easy-to-see diagram of the eye to impress you with, but alas! I ran out of gas. If you're charged up and ready for an anatomy exam, here are a couple of sites that have *great* diagrams:

en.wikipedia.org/wiki/Human_eye

en.wikipedia.org/wiki/Globe_(human_eye)

Cornea: This functions as a shield and as a type of lens. It covers and protects the aqueous humor, the iris and the pupil, and helps to focus incoming light.

Aqueous humor: After light passes through the cornea, it travels through a clear, watery fluid called the aqueous humor. This clear fluid between the cornea and the iris circulates throughout the front part of the eye, maintaining a constant pressure there.

Iris and pupil: The iris is the colored part of

the eye, which contains the dark pupil in its center. The pupil is the opening that light passes through to reach the retina. The pupil contracts and expands as needed to regulate the amount of light that reaches the retina.

Lens: After light travels through the pupil, it passes through the lens. The lens of the human eye, much like the lens of a camera, is responsible for focusing light to create an image. In the eye, the lens focuses the light on the retina, rather than on photographic film.

Vitreous humor, or vitreous: After being focused by the lens, light passes through the center of the eye on its way to the retina. The vitreous, a clear, jellylike substance, fills much of the internal space of the eye and maintains the eye's spherical shape. The vitreous also holds the retina in place along the back wall of the eye.

Retina: The retina is thin, light-sensitive tissue that lines the back of the eye, acting much like film in a camera. Light must be properly focused onto the retina, and the surface of the retina must be flat, smooth, and in good working order to produce a clear image.

Macula: This is the center or bull's-eye of the retina, which contains a high concentration of cone photoreceptor cells that are capable of distinguishing color.

Choroid: This layer of blood vessels behind the retina supplies oxygen and nutrients to the outer layers of the retina.

Sclera: The white part of the eye is called the sclera. It's made up of tough, fibrous tissue that protects the inner workings of the eye.

Optic Nerve: This is a bundle of nerve fibers that carry visual information from the retina to the brain.

More about the retina

When light reaches the retina, it is converted into electrical-chemical signals by the rod and cone photoreceptor cells (*photoreceptor* means "light-receiving"), which are supported by the retinal pigment epithelium. Damage to or degeneration of the rods, cones, or epithelial cells will cause vision problems, which is essentially what happens in inherited retinal degenerative diseases.

Rod photoreceptor cells are essential for night vision, peripheral vision and detecting movement. When I say night, I mean pure darkness with no moon or artificial light. Rods are extremely sensitive to light. These are the cells that die off first in retinitis pigmentosa.

Cone photoreceptor cells detect color and mediate high visual acuity. Cones are crucial to our central vision. Macular degeneration and other diseases that affect the central vision are caused by damage to cone photoreceptor cells.

The **retinal pigment epithelium** (RPE) is located beneath the retina. It absorbs excess light, transports nutrients and removes cellular wastes from the photoreceptor cells. A healthy RPE is essential to having healthy retinal cells; an unhealthy RPE will cause problems such as wet and/or dry age-related macular degeneration.

After light is processed by the retina into electrical-chemical signals, the information is sent to the brain via the optic nerve. Because the eye (and therefore, the retina) is part of the central nervous system, research about other neurodegenerative central nervous system diseases such as Parkinson's and Alzheimer's disease may have applications to retinal degenerative diseases (and vice versa).

The day I received my diagnosis, the observing doctors were talking amongst themselves — about me. They used a word that I hadn't heard, *scotoma.* As Dr. Fishman was performing his exam that word scotoma was resonating harshly in my head. I thought, Cancer! In the case of retinal disease, scotomas are the "blind spots" in our field of vision. Essentially these are areas with no photoreceptors (so no light passes through).

Visual Acuity and What 20/20 Means

Most people think about sight or vision according to the Snellan eye chart at an optometrist's office, which is supposed to measure *visual acuity*. According to the online *Webster's New World Dictionary*, visual acuity is defined as "the ability of the eye to discriminate detail." Visual acuity describes your central vision, but as I discuss later, it does not measure or diagnose the sorts of vision problems that most people who have retinal degenerative diseases experience.

The Snellan eye chart consists of 11 rows of *supposedly* high-contrast (dark black on bright white) letters and numbers, which vary in size from very large in the top row (row 1), to very small in the bottom row (row 11). Each row of the chart has a fraction next to it, such as 20/20, 20/30, 20/40, etc. The largest letter, the E at the top of the chart, has 20/200 next to it.

The fractions relate to the ability to identify objects from a specified distance, which is 20 feet, represented by the numerator (the upper number) of the fraction. The standard for describing normal visual acuity is 20/20, meaning that the average person standing 20 feet from the chart can easily read the 20/20 row (the eighth row in the chart).

The bottom number of the fraction (the denominator) is based on the 20/20 standard. That is, the average human eye can see the eighth row (20/20) from a distance of 20 feet. All the other rows represent exceptions to that standard. The rows above 20/20 are 20/25, 20/30, 20/40, 20/50, 20/70, 20/100 and 20/200. If you cannot read the 20/20 row, but can accurately read the 20/40 row, it means that your visual acuity is *worse than the average*. Your eyes see a high-contrast object from 20 feet away that the "average" person can see from 40 feet away. Of course, if you can accurately read the rows that are *below* the 20/20 row, it means your visual acuity is *better than the average* – you can see high-contrast objects from 20 feet that the average person can only see from 10 or 5 feet.

The problem with this standardized method of measuring visual acuity is that it provides little information about seeing large objects or objects with poor contrast. Nor does it measure how much effort is needed to see clearly.

In short, the visual-acuity test measures only the smallest details that we can see with our central vision; it does not measure our peripheral vision or the quality of our vision. As I discussed in the chapter about how difficult it was for me to get the right diagnosis, most of my eye doctors struggled to diagnose me using visual-acuity testing and corrective lenses. It wasn't until Dr. Kraff realized that my eyesight wasn't correctable using those tools that he referred me to specialists who figured out I had cone-rod dystrophy.

If your visual acuity is considered to be 20/200 or worse, and can't be corrected with eyeglasses, you should be referred to an ophthalmologist who will conduct a low-vision examination. In this case, you may have a whole battery of tests that might include contrast-sensitivity tests, light-sensitivity tests, and electroretinograms (ERGs). Although these are anxiety-provoking and nerve-wracking tests to take, they are the best way to figure out what's causing your vision problems if you have a retinal disease. I am pleased to say that the testing is becoming less and less invasive, and more and more accurate.

Human Genetics — the Basics

Because most retinal degenerative diseases are caused by genetic mutations that are inherited, it's good to know a little about human genetics in order to understand your disease, its possible treatments, and what research is being done.

You'll be happy to know that I took it upon myself to do *"a little"* research on this subject. Hopefully, I have distilled the most important aspects of basic genetics into a form that is understandable. Most of my information came from conversations with medical doctors and researchers.

Chromosomes, genes and DNA

At conception, a fertilized human egg receives 23 chromosomes from the female parent and 23 chromosomes from the male parent. The chromosomes are made from DNA, which contains all the information that enables a fertilized human egg to grow into a fetus, and continue growing and changing into a child, teenager, adult, old person, etc. (DNA is the building block for every part of our cells, but for our purposes we'll concentrate on chromosomes and genes.) Every cell in your body contains a complete set of your chromosomal DNA.

There are 23 pairs of chromosomes in every cell of the body. Twenty-two of the pairs are considered autosomes (non-sex chromosomes) and the 23rd pair are sex chromosomes, consisting of either an X and a Y if you are a male and two X chromosomes if you are a female.

Each chromosome contains thousands of genes, which are individual pieces of genetic information. Most of your genes are like those of every other person on the planet, but about 1 percent of your genes are different from everyone else's (unless you're an identical twin, and then every gene is the same). These are mostly the genes that control traits — for example, the color of your hair, its texture, the shape of your nose, your height, your eye color, eye shape, and even the interior structure of your eyes. For example, myopia and astigmatism are inherited eye conditions.

Similarly, retinal degenerative diseases are inherited eye conditions that are generally caused by mutations in various genes. A gene mutation is a permanent change in the DNA sequence that makes up a gene. Mutations range in size from a single DNA building block (DNA base) to a large segment of a chromosome. Gene mutations can be harmless – for example, the different eye colors, skin colors and hair colors that people have are the result of non-disease-causing mutations called polymorphisms. But they can also be harmful if they change how an organ (such as your retina) develops and behaves.

Gene mutations occur in two different ways. They can be inherited from a parent or occur during a person's lifetime. We will focus on the former – mutations that are inherited.

Mutations that are passed from parent to child at the time of conception (from the female's or the male's chromosomes) are called hereditary mutations. In rare instances, *both* parents carry a gene mutation for a disease that is passed along to a child. This is the case in cystic fibrosis and most retinal degenerative diseases.

Trying to understand genetics and chance

After I was diagnosed with cone-rod dystrophy, my good friend Joanna Zeiger, an epidemiologist and athlete, refreshed my memory of the Punnett square during a long plane ride to a race in Hawaii. Although she was delighted to help me, I couldn't help but feel how difficult it was for her to reduce this information to lay terms. Fortunately for me, she was very patient.

Like me, in high school you probably were taught how to make Punnett squares to determine the probabilities of obtaining a pink-eyed fly if you crossed a white-eyed fly with a red-eyed fly. (Instead of frying your brain with that old lesson, I'll refer to the relatively simple human trait of eye color.

You may recall the AA, Aa, aA, and aa genotypes that the Punnett square describes. Remember, we receive _two_ sets of chromosomes, one set from Mom and one set from Dad. That means you get two genes for every trait, such as your eye color. An individual member of this set of two genes is called an *allele.* An allele from Mom and an allele from Dad combine to create each trait. Some alleles are *dominant,* meaning that the trait they describe will "win" over another allele. For example, with eye color, the allele for brown eyes is dominant and the allele for blue eyes is *recessive.* If you received an allele for brown eyes and an allele for blue eyes, you'd have brown eyes. Only if you received two alleles for blue eyes would your eyes be blue.

In the Punnett square, the capital A represents the dominant allele, and the lower-case A is the recessive allele. In most cases (AA, Aa and aA), the dominant allele will express the trait (as in the brown versus blue eyes example, above); but in one case (aa), the recessive trait will be expressed. See anthro.palomar. edu/mendel_2.htm for Punnett squares, if you haven't had "enough, already!" Below is the Punnet sqare:

	A	a
A	AA	Aa
a	Aa	aa

There are four major patterns of genetic inheritance: autosomal recessive, autosomal dominant, and X-linked recessive and dominant. Remember, *autosomal* means that the genetic material is *not* on the X or Y chromosomes (the "sex" chromosomes). X-linked means that the genetic material is found only on the X sex chromosome.

Autosomal recessive genetic inheritance accounts for approximately 70 percent of inherited retinal disease. Recessive diseases tend to show up in one generation and then disappear for several generations. When a recessive disease shows up in a family where the parents do not have the disease, it means that each parent has one normal allele and one mutated allele. Please note that an allele is a form of a gene and quite often the terms "alleles" and "genes" can be used interchangeably. You can think of each parent as having the genotype Bb. The Punnett square analysis predicts that each time two carrier parents (Bb and Bb) reproduce, there will be a 25 percent chance they will have a child who has the genotype bb — that is, *each time* those parents reproduce, there is a 25 percent chance that the resulting child will inherit two mutated genes and therefore will have the recessive disease.

Autosomal dominant inherited disease accounts for about 20 percent of all inherited retinal disease. In contrast to recessively inherited disease that shows up in just one generation, dominantly inherited disease is a multigenerational disease in which children, parents, aunts, uncles and grandparents may be affected. With dominant inherited disease, only one parent carries a single copy of the mutated gene. There is a 50 percent chance that the mutated gene (and the disease) will be passed along to *any child* of that parent.

X-linked recessive is the least common inheritance pattern, accounting for about 10 percent of retinal diseases. Briefly, in X-linked disease, the mutated gene resides on the X chromosome. Because the mutated gene normally is not expressed if there's a healthy version of the gene on another X chromosome, females, who have two X chromosomes (XX), are less likely to have X-linked disease than males, who have only one X chromosome (XY). Females who have one X chromosome with the mutated gene and one without the mutated gene normally do not get the disease, but can pass the mutation to male children. The best example of this trait is in situations of red-green colorblindness. It is said that 7 to 10 percent of males inherit this trait, while only 1 percent of females inherit the red-green colorblindness trait. The probabilities and genetics of X-linked inheritance are so complex that I recommend discussing it with a specialist if you have an X-linked retinal disease or just want to learn more about the topic.

Confused yet? Read on and then seek further

information from online Web sites or your doctors. The questions never stop for me! My dad says, "It's just a matter of math," but I still believe it is more complicated than that. I encourage you to do your own research if you feel you need more detail. Although I did my best to write this as clearly as possible, I know my explanation isn't perfect. I do feel that I have hit the general ideas and am close to being accurate.

Hopeful Therapies

There are a number of new therapies that treat genetic diseases by going to the source — that is, by treating the disease at the DNA level. Here's a brief discussion of some therapies that may be useful in treating RDDs, perhaps within the next few years.

Gene therapy

Gene therapy is the insertion of normal genes into an individual's cells and tissues to treat a disease, such as a hereditary disease in which a damaging mutated allele is replaced with a functional one. Gene therapy can also be used for human genetic enhancement, changing one's genetic formula and function towards a desired goal of "enhancement." Although the technology is still in its infancy, it has been used with some success, and scientific break-throughs continue to move gene therapy to-wards mainstream medicine. For retinal de-generative disease, gene therapy might mean replacing a mutated gene that causes retinal disease with a functioning "normal" gene. This is our hope, anyway! As you will read below, The Children's Hospital in Philadelphia has made huge breakthroughs in gene therapy. I encourage you all to follow these studies and clinical trials, as their progress is exciting.

Cell-based (stem cell) therapies

This is the area that I am least comfortable writ-ing about, but not for moral or ethical reasons. Stem cell therapy is a highly technical field, and I know very few people who can explain it to the layman. However, I am told by doctors that this therapy offers the most hope for regrowing damaged or lost retinal tissue that contains photoreceptor cells. I consulted the National Institutes of Health (NIH) for much of my research on this topic, and suggest you do the same if you want to learn more.

Stem cells are the most basic of our body's cells. They are responsible for creating and repairing systems, and they are able to become any type of specialized cell. I don't understand how they become specialized, but at some point stem cells change from being nonspecific (having the potential of being a red blood cell or an eye cell or a liver cell) to being fully committed to being a certain type of organ cell. Stem cells are found in your bone marrow, your skin, and in embryos. When used therapeutically, stem cells can repair damage and stop diseases. You can think of stem cells as an internal repair system.

There is so much to learn about this subject, such as the differences between embryonic stem cells and adult stem cells, and how scientists harvest stem cells from skin. I think our community needs to be very open and supportive of stem cell therapy. It is *extremely* important for treating and possibly curing diseases such as Parkinson's, Alzheimer's, leukemia and many of the retinal diseases. Using a single cell to grow into many different types of cells to repair damaged or lost cells is a spectacular and hopeful development.

In fact, as I write this, a company called Advanced Cell Technologies (A.C.T.) just announced a breakthrough in their stem cell treatment for Stargardt's macular dystrophy. This will give hope to those who have cone-rod and rod-cone dystrophy, as all these diseases share the same gene mutation. Of course, this also gives us hope for *all* retinal degenerative diseases. It is naïve to think that treating one of these diseases will not lead to treating another!

It is unclear if the A.C.T. therapy will fix photo-receptor cells; however, it is a step in the right direction. Once again, please ask your specialist about the differences. It is important for the lay person to understand the distinctions. A.C.T. was hoping to move forward with the Phase I clinical trial in early 2010. (*To learn more about the various phases and qualification of clinical trials, visit the U. S. National Institutes of Health at http://clinicaltrials.gov/ ct2/info/understand.*)

Where Are We in Finding Treatments and Cures?

When I read over my own words and the stories in this book, I imagine your response: "Thank you for sharing these inspirational stories, Michael. I feel better about my disease, and inspired to go out and live like the people in your book — but what I really want to know is: Is there any hope for cures or treatments? And if there is, when will they happen?"

I am right there with you! A few years back I

was at a blindness research conference when a gentleman (who was being honored for his fundraising efforts) suggested that researchers' time-frame estimates should be given in "dog years." Although the researchers there may have cringed, I thought his statement was hilarious — and also very real. I am sure many people reading this book can relate to hearing the promise, "There should be treatments or cures in the next five years." Then five years come and go and there's still no treatment or cure, and we feel more helpless than ever.

That being said, there is more hope for results from specific blindness research than ever before. As I write this chapter, I know of at least seven clinical trials that are advancing. There is more promise for our cause right now than at any other time. I assure you that I couldn't have said that five years ago.

In 2009, young adults blind from LCA were able to read from an eye chart and navigate around an obstacle course after undergoing new procedures. This gives us great reason to hope for some progress, and soon! At the time of writing (June 2010), the LCA study at the Children's Hospital in Philadelphia has had dramatic breakthroughs and continues to make enormous progress. I am told that several of the people in the program have been able to put away their walking canes!

Recently, I read a news report of a young American girl living in Denver who went through stem cell treatments in China and just passed her driver's exam. However, researchers have told me that no papers on these Chinese treatments have yet been published in reputable medical journals. I am certain a simple online search could tell you more.

Although the U.S. and other countries have lost much time in the area of stem cell research, it seems to be the greatest hope for re-growing and repairing retinal tissue. I say "seems" because, as you will see below, there are several other fantastic advancements that are also very close to alternative forms of treatments and cures.

I can't tell anyone how he or she should view their responsibility to the larger community. It is even more difficult to tell people who struggle with vision loss that they need to put effort into helping researchers do their jobs by funding their programs. I say this especially for those who have already lost their vision and have adjusted to their condition. Why should they work on behalf of finding a cure? For example, Gordon Gund is a person who won't directly benefit from supporting vision research; he has already lost his vision, and thankfully his children don't have an RDD. So why does he work so hard at finding a cure? Why do the thousands that support organizations like the Foundation Fighting Blindness continue their fundraising efforts? Do we have a responsibility to others with RDD — both those already alive and those yet to be born — who *will eventually* have struggles similar to our own?

I hope most of you will respond with a definitive "*yes!*" At the very least, we need to support the doctors who do this research for little or no financial reward. As far as I am concerned, this is as close to altruism as can be. The problem is, if we don't support their efforts, than we will lose these wonderful researchers, and the hope for cures will be lost, too. Do we really want more people to needlessly suffer? Of course we don't – it's a silly statement.

When you do an Internet search on RDDs, you'll find that there are few charities or foundations anywhere in the world that fight these diseases. You'll find conflicting information. And you'll find there are very few doctors with expertise in the subject. Even the best ophthalmologists and retina specialists have difficulty diagnosing these diseases. The doctors who can make accurate diagnoses are few and far between. We can't afford to lose them, with or without new research. I suffered my whole life from vision problems, and didn't know the cause until I was in my 30s. If more doctors were better informed about RDDs and how to diagnose them, or when to refer patients to specialists, that kind of delay and suffering could be avoided.

The good news is that there *is* in fact hope, and for the most part RDD research is way ahead of research for other inherited diseases. Ironically, blindness-related diseases have the most possibility and promise for cures, but are some of the least funded.

What follows is a brief description of companies that are conducting current research programs and have future plans for clinical trials. For the most up-to-date information, visit the Foundation Fighting Blindness' Web site at www.blindness.org. If you don't find what you're looking for, contact FFB directly. That's what they are there for!

Neurotech: Their treatment shows promise in clinical trials for RP and AMD. Neurotech has just announced encouraging results from their two FFB-funded Phase II/III clinical studies of encapsulated cell technology (ECT) for the treatment of retinitis pigmentosa, Usher's syndrome, and choroideremia.

At the 12-month point in both of those studies, retinas that received high-dose treatments appeared thicker, and likely healthier, than those untreated or receiving low-dose treatments. While that has not yet translated into improved vision, both studies continue to move forward. One trial is an 18-month investigation for people with late-stage disease. The other study is a 30-month investigation for early-stage disease.

In a corporate press release it was reported in March of 2009, the ECT showed good results in a 12-month Phase II study for people with geographic atrophy (dry age-related macular degeneration). The ECT stabilized vision in 96.3 percent of people who received a high dose of the treatment, and Neurotech is planning a Phase III study of the treatment.

Applied Genetic Technologies Corporation (AGTC): A clinical-stage gene therapy development company, AGTC announced it has raised $11.8 million in venture capital funding to advance treatments for Leber's congenital amaurosis and achromatopsia. It is also developing gene therapies for retinoschisis and wet age-related macular degeneration (AMD).

Oxford BioMedica: This company is a key partner of the FFB's clinical trial support organization, the National Neurovision Research Institute. Oxford BioMedica has established a partnership with Sanofi-Aventis, a major international pharmaceutical company, to develop and commercialize gene therapy treatments for Stargardt's disease, Usher's syndrome, and age-related macular degeneration. Based on the agreement, Oxford BioMedica will receive an upfront payment of $26 million and a further $24 million from Sanofi-Aventis over a three-year period. This partnership is a wonderful boost for the development of promising gene therapies.

Approximately half of all cone-rod dystrophies are caused by mutations in the *ABCA-4 gene, the same gene responsible for Stargardt's disease. We hope that a treatment for the Stargardt's gene will work for cone-rod dystophy.

According to FFB's Dr. Tim Schoen, "I think that one of the most exciting potential treatments for ABCA-4 mediated disease is the ABCA-4 lentiviral gene therapy being developed by Dr. Allikmets and Oxford Biomedica."

Sirion Therapeutics: Although this company is no longer in existence, having been acquired by Alcon, they were developing a drug called Fenretinide, which slowed the progression of advanced dry age-related macular degeneration by 45 percent in people receiving a high-dose treatment in a Phase II clinical trial. Oth-

---

* According to Joanna Zeiger, Ph.D., all genes have genetic and genomic nomenclature. This has been established by the HUGO Gene Nomenclature Committee or HGNC for each known human gene in the form of an approved gene name and given a symbol or short-form abbreviation. All approved symbols are stored in their database. Each symbol is unique, and each gene is given only one approved gene symbol. It is necessary to provide a unique symbol for each gene in an effort to discuss it properly. Each disease that I have discussed has a specific gene name, but there are hundreds of variations. For example, retinitis pigmentosa has several different gene names to describe the specific form that a person might have.

er companies such as Acucela are developing similar therapies for Stargardt's disease and dry age-related macular degeneration.

FFB funded early, preclinical studies of Fenretinide, which demonstrated the drug's potential for slowing vision loss in people affected by mutations in the ABCA-4 gene. I am hopeful that Sytera, the company that originally developed Fenretinide, will take over the oversight of the trials so as not to lose any time.

Pfizer: The giant pharmaceutical company announced a major investment in embryonic stem cell research for age-related macular degeneration taking place at University College London. Researchers hope to begin a clinical study of the stem cell treatment in two years. Pfizer's financial backing and clinical and commercial expertise greatly strengthens the potential for stem cells to be used as a treatment for AMD in the near future.

Mitochondria: A Potential Treatment for Retinal Degeneration and Other Disease?

It has been a privilege to read the reports and hear the various presentations about the research noted above. It has also been fascinating to learn more about new research entering the field of vision restoration.

In February 2010 I attended the Foundation Fighting Blindness' Day of Science, something I participate in annually. We have the opportunity to meet with the world's top doctors and researchers in the field of retinal degenerative disease. However, I have to highlight one presentation that caught my attention in a profound manner. The presenter was Dr. Baerbel (Barb) Rohrer, Ph.D., from the University of South Carolina. As I sat taking notes, attempting to understand, Dr. Rohrer spoke of ATP (adrenosine triphosphate). When I heard that word my ears perked up and I had to make certain I was hearing her correctly. I will discuss the specifics of this below, but the reason her words caught my attention is that ATP and the whole bio-energetic process is part of my everyday language as an athlete, coach and personal trainer. Was I now hearing that this system could be a potential treatment or cure for RDDs? I had often sat in my exercise physiology classes listening to lectures on ATP and fantasizing that this concept could be applied to photoreceptor cell regeneration. Of course, it was just a fantasy — or was it?

The neurons of the retina require large amounts of adenosine triphosphate; it is the universal energy currency of all living organisms. The majority of ATP is produced in cellular organelles (a specialized sub-unit of a cell) called mitochondria. ATP requires simple and complex sugars (carbohydrates) or lipids (fats) as an energy source. However, mitochondrial function and ATP production are very sensitive to environmental challenges, as well as aging. Tissues from elderly patients show a decrease in ATP production. Dr. Rohrer and her partner Craig Beeson have shown in preliminary experiments that they can utilize existing FDA-approved drugs to keep photoreceptor cells healthy. They further hypothesize that changes in cellular metabolism may be a major factor in retinal degenerative disease, and that manipulation of cellular metabolism may provide novel and promising therapeutic approaches to the treatment of retinal degeneration. Who would have thought that the *energy* could be the cure to many diseases? What makes this treatment even more exciting is that using existing FDA-approved drugs will dramatically accelerate the process of moving from the drug discovery state to human clinical trials.

I find this all particularly exciting, as I am told that photoreceptor cells have more mitochondria than *any* other part of the body! If it has already worked in the lab — this noninvasive research is very promising.

As with all the existing clinical trials and potential therapies noted above, please visit FFB's Web site for up-to-date information.

eye envy

chapter 16

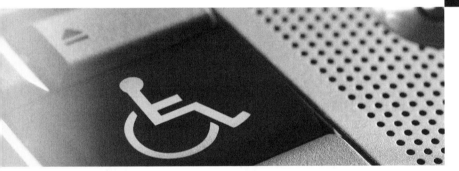

ADA made simple

What is it and what does it mean for us?

I first became involved with ADA compliance issues as a hotel/resort owner and developer. This was well before I had any idea what was awaiting me with my own vision loss. I took the matter very seriously. I went well beyond what was considered "compliance." The laws are written in a general way in order to apply to many different situations, and this unfortunately leaves a rather large door open for interpretation. Most of us go about our day and never notice the hardships of people who have disabilities; many people simply turn their heads with pity. I recall one encounter when I was in my own resort well after we made our ADA enhancements. I was in an elevator with a man in a wheelchair. As he entered the elevator, the door closed on him even with me holding the door open. I was thankful that I could actually correct this problem and began to wonder what else I could do. Please keep in mind that I was only thinking of those in wheelchairs. I knew we had audio solutions for the hearing impaired. As for the visually impaired, I thought the Braille placards would suffice.

Oddly enough, I never considered the visually impaired. Of course, my perspective has changed! Now I walk into a restaurant and can't see the dimly colored menu posted on a wall seven feet away. When I ask for a printed menu, the typeface is so small and has such poor contrast, I have to ask someone to read it to me. Finding my way through an airport is even worse. Airports could be improved if the "powers that be" simply thought of lighting, contrast, the position of the signage, and the type size. Improvements would not be costly. I have every intention of taking it upon myself to consult an attorney to help us overcome such problems. Clearly, the airport scenario is remedied by the fact that airports employ many people who are there to assist people who need help. That said, I am able to move through an airport by asking for minor help here and there. I have no desire to use one of those employees who are provided for the specific purpose of helping disabled individuals. I would rather they assist people in greater need than I.

I am not certain why all the street signs are of low contrast, but it would be interesting to hear the reasoning. Of course, it all begins to make sense when you read the "undue hardship" clause in the ADA document as a metaphoric "get out of jail free" card. Think about the shocking, huge expense it would take to change some signs! When physical improvements are being made, such as in signage or lighting, responsible decision makers should go one step further. That's my personal feeling, and one that I will seek an answer to. Most certainly, anything that assists the visually impaired will also help the fully sighted.

It was not until recently that I started to seek out special seating for concerts, shows and sports events. *Most* of the time the so-called special seating is downright offensive. My sister-in-law and I recently went to see a U2 concert in Chicago. We paid top dollar for what we were told were "visually accessible" seats from which we could "easily see the performance." When we arrived, we realized that there were no special seats for us and we couldn't have been further from the stage. Even worse, there was a pole obstructing what poor view we had. We then had to deal with the embarrassment of asking for help. We missed the entire first set. We also realized that what the venue really meant by "visually accessible" was that all disabled people, no matter what their disability, would be seated together. So we sat with the people who were in wheelchairs. The truth is, I felt just as bad for them as I did for us.

For many, disabled is disabled and it doesn't matter what the disability is. This is not the case everywhere, and we do have rights. But it's up to us to seek out these rights and make the most of our challenges. Yes, it's frustrating and time consuming. Once again, we hope the end will justify the means.

I spoke of attorneys. I am not a litigious person and feel very strongly that we should not make litigation our first remedy. But I do feel that *anyone* with a disability is justified in seeking appropriate legal counsel in an effort to further define our rights, and also to show the general public what can be done to make disabled people's lives easier.

Fortunately for us, we have a good friend and champion, who is featured in this book. This is Jeremy Block. He has helped me find the resources to provide you with the information below. I did my very best, much like in the Science section, to make this as easy to understand as possible. Don't forget to consult professionals with specific questions. You might just find that your concerns have already been addressed.

So, what is the ADA?

Often described as the most sweeping anti-discrimination legislation since the Civil Rights Act of 1964, the Americans with Disabilities Act of 1990 (ADA) provides broad legal protections in employment, public services, public accommodations, services operated by public entities, and transportation for people who have disabilities. The act's stated purpose is "to provide a clear and comprehensive national mandate for the elimination of discrimination against individuals with disabilities." Please visit this site for greater detail: http://frwebgate.access.gpo.gov/cgi-bin/usc.cgi?ACTION=BROWSE&TITLE=42USCC126&PDFS=YES).

The concept of providing protections for people with disabilities is not new. The ADA is based on Section 504 of the Rehabilitation Act of 1973. This law prohibits discrimination against people who have disabilities, or because of their disabilities, by any program of the federal government or by any entity that receives federal funding.

Historically, people with disabilities have faced challenges when living amongst the general population while attempting to achieve the "great American dream." Typically, these challenges are due to societal barriers rather than to the nature of the disability. These difficulties include living in the community or working next to people without disabilities, gaining access to the same venues as people without disabilities, and using technology in the same fashion as people without disabilities. The purpose of the ADA is to remove these artificial barriers imposed by society and ensure that people with disabilities are not discriminated against.

The ADA has five distinct sections, called titles. The section that generally receives the most attention is Title I. Title I covers the responsibilities employers must meet when hiring and providing accommodations to current or potential employees with disabilities.

Specifically, Title I prohibits discrimination against a person with a disability on the basis of that disability in regard to job application procedures; the hiring, advancement or firing of employees; compensation; job training; and other conditions of employment. Antidiscrimination provisions in Title I of the ADA are specifically for "qualified" people with disabilities or "an individual with a disability who, with or without reasonable accommodation, can perform the essential functions (duties and responsibilities) of the employment position that such person holds or desires."

As stated above, Title I of the ADA requires employers to provide reasonable accommodation to assist a person with a disability in fulfilling the duties of a position. "Reasonable accommodation" is defined in the ADA as making existing facilities readily accessible to and usable by people with disabilities.

Reasonable accommodations may include job restructuring, modified work schedules, reassignment to a vacant position, acquisition of assistive technology, modification of equipment or devices, and adjustment of examinations or training materials or policies, to name a few. For example, a person who is blind or visually impaired may be qualified for a position but may need to use a screen reader to meet the essential functions of the position. The employer's purchase of the screen reader in response to the employee or potential employee's request would a reasonable accommodation.

However, providing reasonable accommodations cannot cause undue hardship for the employer. "Undue hardship" is defined as "an action requiring significant difficulty or expense." For example, a person with low vision recently hired at a nightclub may request as a reasonable accommodation the installation of lights behind the bar in order to see bottles and denominations on currency better. An employer may deny the request based on undue hardship — lighting installation may be expensive. Additionally, the installation of the lights may also undermine the inherent nature of the employment site, which includes a dimly lit atmosphere. The employer must work with the employee on finding alternatives, such as specific self-lighting accessories or other more suitable accommodations.

Title II of the ADA prohibits discrimination by state and local government agencies. Specifically, the law states that no individual with a disability shall be excluded from participation in or be denied the benefits of the services, programs or activities of a state, local government or public entity. Public entities include public authorities or commissions established for a public purpose or conducted by or on behalf of the government.

The Department of Justice, which has a responsibility to ensure fair and impartial administration of justice for all Americans, has developed guidance or regulations for Title II on accessibility. Each service, program or activity conducted by a government or public entity must be readily accessible to and usable by individuals with disabilities. This access includes physical access – being able to enter or maneuver inside of public entities – and programmatic access – access to programs. Most people understand physical access. It includes ramps for gaining access to buildings, Braille signage in elevators, and emergency lights in buildings that have both visual indicators (a flash) and auditory indicators (a siren or an announcement). Governments and public entities are not required to make each of their existing facilities accessible.

Programmatic accessibility assures that governments and public entities policies and practices do not hinder the ability of the person with a disability to receive the same services as other persons. For example, a public housing commission may host a public forum in a privately owned building in which they rent office space. The building may have a "no pets" policy; however, programmatic accessibility in the ADA allows individuals with service or support animals to enter the premises. But programmatic accessibility has its limitations too. A public entity is not required to take any action that would result in fundamentally altering its service, program or activity or cause undue financial burdens.

Finally, Title II contains requirements for public transportation other than by aircraft or certain rail operations. All new vehicles purchased or leased by a government or public entity that operates a fixed route system, such as a bus route, must be accessible. Paratransit services must also be provided by the government or public entity that operates a fixed-route service. Rail systems must have at least one car per train that is accessible to individuals with disabilities. Clearly, transportation is an enormous issue for people who cannot drive because of a disability.

Under Title III, people cannot be discriminated against on the basis of a disability from enjoying the goods, services, facilities or accommodations of any public place. Title III covers public accommodations, commercial facilities, and private entities including hotels, restaurants, laundromats, museums, day care centers, physicians' offices and gymnasiums, to name a few. Religious institutions and privately controlled clubs are not included on the list. Whether the ADA applies to Internet sites' accessibility is still being debated.

Title III's nondiscrimination requirements and limitations are similar to those of Titles I and II. Title III discusses architecture that creates physical access barriers but does not have to be modified if the changes cannot be accomplished or carried out without great difficulty or expense.

Title IV of the ADA establishes a national tele-communications relay service and mandates that public-service announcements that are provided or funded in whole or in part by any federal agency be closed-captioned. Title IV is enforced by the Federal Communications Commission.

Finally, Title V contains several provisions applying to all other titles of the ADA. Among other requirements, Title V requires federal agencies to develop technical assistance plans for entities that must comply with the law. It contains a report on wilderness areas and individuals with disabilities, and encourages the use of alternative dispute resolution (ADR). Once again, visit http://www.adata.org/what-sada-structure.aspx for more information on these titles.

Again, should you find these rights unclear or seek further information, please consult an attorney who has specific ADA knowledge.

eye envy

chapter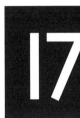

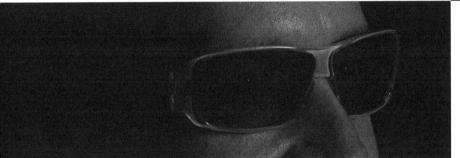

wrap up

Eyewear and Helpful Hints

I hope you have enjoyed what you have read, and that you have gained some degree of hope and new knowledge about retinal degenerative disease. Although none of the people featured in this book know one another, I felt as though their stories shared a common theme. I will leave you to your own conclusions about that. If you are affected by vision loss, I hope that at the very least you were able to relate to what has been shared with you. I can't express enough gratitude to you for taking the time to read this book. Should you desire additional information, please visit my Web site at www.steppingstonesports.com.

How Do We Protect Our Peepers?

"Visual impairments are also genetic reasons to own cool shades!"

It makes sense that those of us who have an RDD should protect what vision we have. I am talking about wearing proper eyewear as well as a hat or visor. I need the best lenses

I can find just to do the sports I do, because glare overwhelms my vision. It took me years to find the lenses that I use, even with sponsorships from most of the major sunglass companies. In fact, that complicated matters because I sometimes used lenses that didn't help my vision just because my sponsoring company recommended them. Not until I met the folks at Zeal Optics and had an appointment with my doctor did I really begin to understand this.

My doctor lectured me on why lens color or tint is important to vision, and not just as protection from the sun's harmful rays, as one might tend to believe. He also discussed light transmission and explained the range of light that should be allowed through my lenses for my vision problems. My doctor suggested I use a lens that has a reddish brown to amber tint, and stay away from blue or grey.

I also needed something that would improve visibility. I randomly brought in several pairs of sunglasses to my doctor and he tested them all for me. To my surprise, the best lenses were also the least expensive of the group! Coincidentally, my friend Jamie Whitmore introduced me to Michael and Wink Jackson, the founders of Zeal Optics, who made those lenses. At the time they were based in Moab, Utah, but they have since moved their small company to my hometown of Boulder. I tried their lenses in many different scenarios and found that they really do work best for me. I am so grateful that they continue to dedicate themselves to making such great eyewear for everyday use as well as sports.

When I asked Michael and Wink to summarize what good lenses should provide, this is what they had to say:

"A sunglass in principle should protect your eyes from the sun's harmful UV rays; protect from flying objects; reduce the glare from the sun; and help you see the best you can."

I asked them about light transmission. "Visual light transmittance, or VLT, is important, but not as important as the lens tint. You can have a VLT of 13 percent in a grey lens and a VLT of our Zeal-blend tint at 13 percent, but they are not the same. Different tints have different effects, such as improved contrast and reduced glare."

When Zeal started making sunglasses 13 years ago, most eyewear companies were focused on image and marketing rather than the performance of the eyewear they offered. Not much has changed since then, with most of these companies still focused on image marketing and smoke and mirrors. Zeal set out to change this. Most people don't pay attention to the tint or color of the lens, but this is one of the most important factors when choosing a sunglass. Zeal's ZB13 lens was engineered to improve vision. It doesn't strain your eyes or distort the colors you see. Most lens tints are grey, brown, orange, blue or green, rather than a blend of tints. This tends to distort the color and make your eyes work harder to see.

UV protection from the sun's harmful rays is also an important consideration in choosing a sunglass. Today, almost every sunglass has this feature.

Author's note: The good news for me was that the Jackson's comments were consistent with what my doctor had told me. Of course you should always ask your own doctor. I have seen way too many people wearing improper eyewear, especially those who should know better! My doctor suggested that I use a tint that is close to amber. I have personally found that this works very well to promote contrast and also results in far less eyestrain. I have experimented with red lenses as well. This idea came to me one day when I was having a "bad vision day." I thought about my photography days and how I used a red filter to promote contrast. I first went to an optometrist and asked him if he could add a red-lens reading glass. He actually used a camera lens for this. As anything with a white or light background is next to impossible for me to see, the red lens worked quite well. I am now experimenting with this concept with Zeal. So far it is working well at times where I am going from light to dark, such as when I am mountain biking or trail running and many shadows exist. It is also nice for indoor conditions where the light is too bright, such as large stores or supermarkets.

Finally, here are a few *one-liners* that were created to make your life just a wee bit easier. Keep them close to both yourself and your heart. This was a collaborative effort between Donna Richards, Jeremy Block and me. We had fun writing them. Some are a bit redundant, but then again, redundancy helps make the point that is intended. At least for me it does!

Donna

"I keep doing things I can't, that's how I get to do them." (a student's paraphrase of a Picasso quote)

"You will always see more with your heart

than your eyes."

"See the person, not the disability."

"It's easier to find things when you look with your mind and not your eyes."

"Put it in your mind's eye."

"Don't let anyone do for you what you can do for yourself — that's the secret to self-empowerment."

"Don't worry about tomorrow. Tomorrow will worry about itself. — Words of encouragement when you get overwhelmed and anxious because everything takes twice as long to do."

Jeremy

"Being visually impaired is just a hurdle, and once you learn proper hurdling technique you can just get over it!"

"Confront stereotypes and misconceptions;

then destroy them by succeeding."

"When you ask me how many fingers you are holding up, all I can see is the same number as your IQ."

"What the eye cannot see, the mind will make up for."

"If Monet was not visually impaired, then how do you explain the blotchy artwork that was a direct reproduction of what he saw?"

"Being visually impaired means you actually feel the music, because we all know none of us can see them playing the instruments."

"Only the visually impaired can see with their ears."

"If someone creates something accessible for a visually impaired person, then it is accessible for everyone. Shouldn't all products be designed that way?"

"Visual impairments are the best argument for

a personal limousine driver."

"Having a visual impairment qualifies you to own the largest television on the market in order to accommodate your disability."

"If you want to be the most fashionable person around, tell a fashionista that you're visually impaired and want them to pick out your wardrobe; they'll do it for free."

"Never wait for someone to figure out what you need. Tell them right away in terms they can understand."

"Give people a chance; happy people are forgiving and flexible."

"Nobody understands what you need better than you."

"When it comes to accommodating your disability, the buck stops with you and nobody else."

"Never underestimate yourself, especially if

someone else clearly has."

"Try it first, then fail, then figure it out, then ask for help, then try it again and succeed."

"Being overprotective is like taking away your body armor."

"The difference between a condescending tone and an assisting tone is whether or not the person believes in you."

"Visual impairments assist in dating because they give you a great excuse to get up close and personal in order to 'see' who someone is."

"Holding the hand of your gorgeous love interest is a wonderful necessity for the visually impaired person walking around in public."

"Visually impaired people are better at dealing with the future. We already know how to handle it when we cannot see what is coming."

Michael

"There is an enormous difference between 'sight' and 'vision.' Who says you must have sight to have vision?"

"Remember, people don't always know that you are visually challenged. Show them as much compassion as you would like them to show you."

"One of the greatest gifts you can give someone else is to allow that someone to help you."

"Remember that your disability is also hard on those who love you."

"You owe your best to those who love you most. Sometimes that love is 'tough love,' but it is still love."

"You will be harder on yourself than others will be on you."

"There's a baby soul in all of us. Every now and again that baby soul requires a little gentle love and needs to be gently rocked to be calm. A little motion goes a long way to calm that soul. Be gentle with yourself."

"A mind's 'eye' is a beautiful thing. The choice is yours as to how you wish to use that mind of yours."

"For you teenagers stressing about your university board tests: Take them untimed! I could have used that advice."

"Fear is a healthy reminder to take one step back and two steps forward."

"Talk to yourself when you feel fear. You will find that voice of yours can be very calming. Try to treat fear not as your enemy, but as your friend that is there to keep you safe."

"Don't be afraid to grieve your loss. Yes, you have lost! But it doesn't mean you have not gained something else in the process."

"Don't ever be afraid to ask for help. Life is challenging enough."

"Keep yourself healthy and fit. You will need all the strength you can get, and life will be so much easier when you are healthy and feeling good."

"You have every right to be 'there,' wherever *there* might take you. Don't ever tell yourself that just because it is a *sighted* world, you don't belong!"

"No one else can define your limitations. If you don't try, who knows what you will accomplish?"

"Don't be afraid to push beyond what you perceive as limitations. You might just find that they were not limitations after all."

"Being visually challenged is an excuse to have permanent beer goggles!".